Manual of Equine Nutrition and Feeding Management

Carol Z. Buckhout, M.P.S., P.A.S.
Barbara E. Lindberg, M.S. Ed.

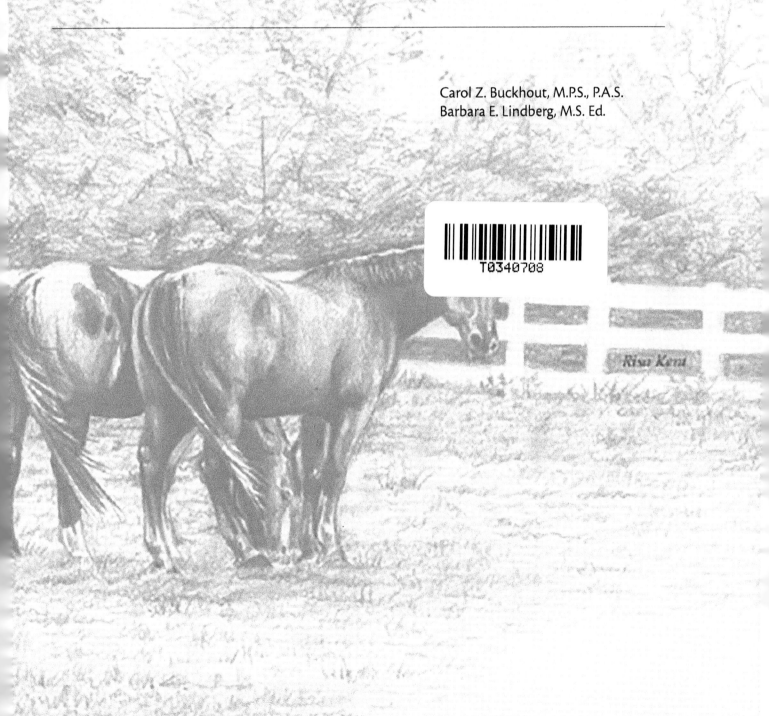

Risa Kent

T0340708

Manual of Equine Nutrition and Feeding Management

First Edition

Authors:

Carol Z. Buckhout, M.P.S., P.A.S.

Professor Emerita

Equine Business Management

Cazenovia College

Barbara E. Lindberg, M.S. Ed.

Associate Professor

Equine Business Management

Cazenovia College

Artwork:

Rachel C. Monticelli-Turner

dobbindesigns@yahoo.com

University of Illinois at Chicago, M.S. Biomedical Visualization, 2008

Cazenovia College B.F.A., 2005

Dutchess Community College, A.A.S. Commercial Art, 2002

Cazenovia College, A.A.S. Equine Studies, 1992

Risa Kent

www.risakent.com

Cazenovia College, B.P.S., 2010

Carmel Keeley

Cazenovia College, B.P.S., 2009

Research Assistant and Text Design:

Sara Tanner Mastellar, Ph.D.

Cazenovia College, B.P.S., 2009

With special thanks to:

Laurie Gilmore Selleck, M.F.A.

Professor

Visual Communications

Cazenovia College

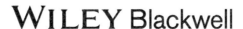

Registered Office
John Wiley & Sons, Inc., 111 River Street, Hoboken, NJ 07030, USA

Editorial Office
111 River Street, Hoboken, NJ 07030, USA

For details of our global editorial offices, customer services, and more information about Wiley products visit us at www. wiley.com.

Wiley also publishes its books in a variety of electronic formats and by print-on-demand. Some content that appears in standard print versions of this book may not be available in other formats.

Library of Congress Cataloging-in-Publication Data Applied for

PB: 9781119063223

Cover Design: Wiley
Cover Images: Timothy grass - James R. Johnson, hosted by the USDA-NRCS PLANTS Database/USDA NRCS. 1992. Western wetland flora: Field office guide to plant species. West Region, Sacramento.
© Scott Sinklier/Design Pics/Getty Images, © Agency Animal Picture/ Getty Images, © Terje Rakke/Getty Images

Set in 10/11pt CronosPro by Straive, Chennai, India

SKY10034273_050222

Dedication

The authors wish to express their sincere appreciation and admiration to the many students of equine nutrition that over the past decades have provided inspiration for the creation of this manual. Their interest and feedback have proved to be invaluable. A special acknowledgement goes to Dr. Sara Tanner Mastellar for her patience and expertise with the numerous re-writes, changes in format and in her spearheading of the Instructors' Companion. The artwork provided by former Cazenovia College students Rachel Monticelli-Turner, Risa Kent, and Carmel Keeley not only enhance the document, but display the versatile talents of Cazenovia College students. Last and most importantly, credit must be given to the beloved horse for, without this magnificent animal, none of our lives would be the same.

Carol Z. Buckhout
Barbara E. Lindberg

TABLE OF CONTENTS

Preface

The suggested use for this manual is in an applied laboratory situation that allows students to have time to explore concepts as well as to work on class activities and assignments. It may serve as a companion document for an equine nutrition lecture course since key topics such as the six classes of nutrients and their functions as well as feeding strategies for various classes of horses are not included. A minimum of a two-hour time period is recommended in order for students to engage in each topic. The organization of the material fits with two key texts: *Feeding and Care of the Horse*, Second Edition, by Lon D. Lewis and *Nutrient Requirements of Horses*, Sixth Revised Edition, by the National Research Council (NRC). Both information and examples provided by Lewis along with nutrient requirements and feed profiles provided by the NRC are useful for completing many of the assignments. While the laboratory concepts and assignments build successively on each other, users of this manual may to choose to omit some labs or their exercises if time becomes a constraint. Alternatively, one may choose to extend the amount of time devoted to certain lab topics, especially Laboratory 1 on digestive anatomy. Assignments are designed to be thought provoking and practical. While answers to some lab questions are succinct, other questions are designed to support the concept that there is both a science and an art to the topic of equine nutrition. The authors acknowledge that there are many ways in which to engage students in the topic of feeding horses, especially now that fewer people have direct ties to production agriculture. The intention for this manual is to combine practical aspects of feeds and feeding along with more technical aspects of equine nutrition. In the end, may it bring our horses continued good health.

Carol Z. Buckhout
Barbara E. Lindberg

Disclaimer

The information in this lab manual was designed to help the horse owner understand practical aspects of equine nutrition and ration balancing. This, however, is only the beginning of understanding equine nutrition. New advances are being made every year, and therefore an astute horse owner will seek to stay current on recent research.

It should also be remembered that consultation with a veterinarian and/or equine nutritionist may be required in some instances. Nutrition should not be viewed as a standalone subject in a vacuum, but as a part of the holistic care of the horse.

About the Companion Website

The companion website for this book is at

www.wiley.com/go/buckhout/manual

The website contains –

An Instructor Site:
- 1–13 Laboratory chapters
- Instructor Answer Key

A Student Site:
- Additional Questions related to Laboratory chapters 1–13

Laboratory 1
THE EQUINE DIGESTIVE SYSTEM

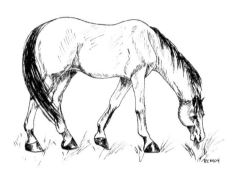

Source: Rachel Monticelli-Turner.

NOTES:

Introduction:

Understanding the anatomical organization and function of the equine digestive system is very important in laying a foundation of knowledge about the nature of feeding horses. In this laboratory exercise the student will review the locations and functions of the organs of digestion, paying particular attention to where the various nutrients are digested and absorbed. This base of knowledge will foster an appreciation for why horses utilize certain types of feeds more efficiently and why horses are prone to various digestive-related disorders.

Objectives:

When finished with the material from this laboratory, the student should be able to:

1. Identify all organs that relate both directly and indirectly to the digestive system of the horse.

2. Define the following terms:
   a. digestion
   b. absorption
   c. metabolism
   d. herbivore
   e. nonruminant
   f. cecal fermenter
   g. ruminant
   h. prehension
   i. mastication
   j. colic
   k. choke.

3. List sizes, capacities, and functions of the organs of the equine digestive tract.

4. List the locations of digestion and absorption for the six classes of nutrients.

Manual of Equine Nutrition and Feeding Management, First Edition.
Carol Z. Buckhout and Barbara E. Lindberg.
© 2022 John Wiley & Sons, Inc. Published 2022 by John Wiley & Sons, Inc.
Companion website: www.wiley.com/go/buckhout/manual

*Ruminant animals
such as cows can digest
quite efficiently by
fermenting feed in a
multi-chambered stomach.
Most nonruminants lack
this fermentation ability
in their foregut, and are
therefore called "simple
stomached". They may
either lack fermentation
ability (like humans and
pigs) or they may be "cecal
fermenters" (like horses)
where fermentation happens
in the hindgut.*

NOTES:

5. Describe the types and arrangement of teeth in the horse's oral cavity and how their shape changes over time. Relate the changes to approximate ages of the horse.

6. Identify similarities and differences of the equine digestive system to both the simple and ruminant digestive systems.

Question for further discussion:

1. Why is the horse prone to digestive disorders such as colic and choke? Suggest feeding strategies that would avoid these situations.

General overview:

As a nonruminant herbivore, the horse is designed to live on a diet of plants, the majority of which are forages. Wild horses graze for 12 to 16 hours per day, consuming small amounts at any one time. Hence, the nature of the horse's digestive tract is to accommodate small, frequent intakes. The horse's teeth wear more evenly and consistently when the animal is able to chew coarse plant material for several hours each day. While the majority of horses on the earth today are no longer wild, they still thrive best when their feeding program is organized to provide small meals, primarily consisting of quality forage, throughout the day.

A thorough understanding of the horse's digestive system is paramount to organizing an appropriate feeding regimen. It also creates the base for understanding why the horse is prone to certain digestive disorders. Keep the size of the mature horse in mind while exploring the numerous organs of digestion, their sizes and their functions throughout this lab.

THE EQUINE DIGESTIVE TRACT: PRIMARY AND SECONDARY ORGANS OF DIGESTION

A. Primary organs of digestion: The upper digestive tract

The following outline provides information pertaining to the primary organs of digestion (feed passes through them) that are considered to be part of the upper digestive tract of the horse. Use this guide when observing the specimens and diagrams provided in the laboratory, but also note there are some areas of the outline intended for the student to complete!

1. **Oral cavity**
   a. *Lips:* well developed and muscular; important tactile properties and involved with prehension of feeds
   b. *Teeth:* involved with prehension and mastication of feeds; deciduous (baby or milk) teeth erupt first and are then replaced by permanent teeth

Figure 1.1 Teeth of an adult horse. *Source: Rachel Monticelli-Turner.*

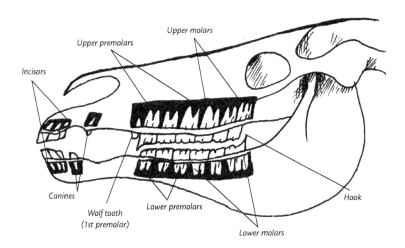

c. Identify each of the following types of teeth (Pence, 2002):

   i. Incisors (I) or front teeth: 6 total (3 per side) on both top and bottom jaws of mature horse, named in pairs for their location: central (I1), intermediate (I2), corner (I3)

   ii. Cheek teeth or grinders:

     1. *Premolars (P):* 6–8 on both top and bottom (3–4 per side), depending on whether wolf teeth are present. They are named for their location; P1, P2, P3, and P4. P1 is also known as the wolf tooth. (More information on wolf teeth can be found on the next page in the sidebar.)

     2. *Molars (M):* 6 on both top and bottom (3 per each side)

   iii. Canines (C): a single canine tooth may be located in the diastema (the space between the incisors and the premolars, also called the bar) and it may be in the top and/or the bottom jaw; canines are more commonly associated with stallions or geldings; a horse might not have any canine teeth or it may have as many as four canines; other names for the canines include: eyeteeth, bridle teeth, tusks, or tushes.

   iv. Parts of the equine tooth (Frandson, Wilke & Fails, 2009): locate each part on specimens or diagrams provided:

     1. root—anchors tooth in its bone socket (alveolus) and is attached to the surrounding bone by periodontium (connective tissue), creating a gomphosis (fibrous) joint

     2. crown—the portion of the tooth above the gum line

     3. neck—the space between crown and root; equine teeth do not have prominent necks and are referred to as hypsodont

---

Dental Formula:

The traditional method for listing the potential number of teeth in a horse is to start with the letter abbreviation of the tooth followed by the number of teeth in the upper jaw placed over the number of teeth in the lower jaw (making it look like a fraction) for half of the horse's head. For example: The total number of incisors for the upper jaw is 6 as well as for the lower jaw. Therefore, the dental formula for only the incisors is:

$$2\left(I\frac{3}{3}\right)=12$$

or 12 total incisors. Deciduous or "baby" teeth are abbreviated with a "D" followed by a lower case letter "i" for incisor or lower case "p" for premolar.

Review the following dental formulas:

Deciduous (milk) teeth

$$2\left(Di\frac{3}{3}, Dp\frac{3}{3}\right)=24$$

Permanent teeth

$$2\left(I\frac{3}{3}, C\frac{0-1}{0-1}, P\frac{3or4}{3or4}, M\frac{3}{3}\right)$$
$$=36-44$$

Figure 1.2 Sagittal section and occlusal surfaces of a permanent lower incisor tooth.
Source: Rachel Monticelli-Turner.

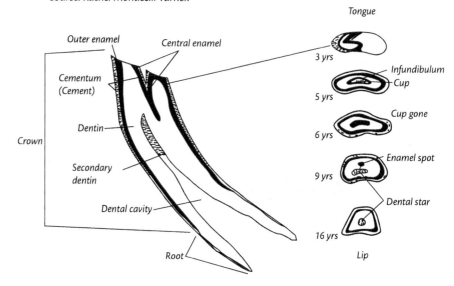

NOTES:

Since mares frequently lack canine teeth they can have as few as 36 teeth.

Wolf teeth—The first premolar, if present, is called the "wolf tooth". These are small vestigial premolars usually found in the upper jaw, but they may also be located in the lower jaw. Their shallow roots allow for a relatively easy removal by a veterinarian. This is often necessary as they will sometimes interfere with the horse's comfort when wearing a bit.

The incisors found in ruminants have a short crown and a more prominent neck than what is found in equines; such teeth are called brachyodont (Frandson, 2003) (Greek: brachy refers to short; hypsi refers to high).

4. dentin—the mineralized substance that comprises most of a tooth's interior; center area called dental cavity contains the dental pulp

5. dental pulp—portion of dental cavity that includes connective tissue, nerves, blood vessels

6. enamel—covers dentin, comprised of inorganic crystals (very hard!); its prominent folds on the grinding surfaces of hypsodont teeth are called cups

7. cementum—thin mineral layer extending from the root and covering the crown of the tooth and filling in the infundibulum of central enamel

8. cup (infundibulum)—the dark central area of the younger tooth created by folds of enamel on grinding surfaces, this may be found on both deciduous and permanent teeth and wears away as the horse ages

9. dental star—this is comprised of the secondary dentin and often first appears as a line in the central incisors, then appears in the intermediate and corner incisors; found on both deciduous and permanent teeth

Aging a horse by its teeth: This was a common practice before the current positive identification systems (tattooing, microchipping, etc.) came into use. It is still useful in determining an approximation of age (Riegel and Hakola, 1999).

Dental Time Line

6 days	*eruption of central deciduous incisors*
Birth–2 wks	*eruption of deciduous premolars 2, 3, and 4*
6 wks	*eruption of intermediate deciduous incisors*
6 mo	*eruption of corner deciduous incisors*
1 yr	*deciduous teeth all present and in wear, central and intermediate incisors have longitudinal dental stars, first permanent premolars may be appearing, central incisor cup disappears with wear; first permanent molars have erupted*
1.5 yrs	*intermediate incisor cup disappears with wear*
2 yrs	*central deciduous incisor is missing in preparation for permanent central incisor, corner incisor cup disappears with wear, corner incisor star visible, second permanent premolar erupts*
2.5 yrs	*eruption of central permanent incisor*
3 yrs	*central incisors erupted and in wear with deep cups, deciduous intermediate and corner incisors appear ready to be replaced, if there are any "wolf teeth" they are seen easily, third permanent premolars erupt*
3.5 yrs	*eruption of intermediate permanent incisor, canines may erupt; third permanent molars have erupted*
4 yrs	*permanent central and intermediate incisors in wear, cups on central incisors are deep, deciduous corner incisors appear small, canines may erupt, fourth permanent premolar erupts*
4.5 yrs	*eruption of corner permanent incisor*
5 yrs	*permanent dentition complete, canines completely erupted, all incisors have cups*
6 yrs	*central incisor permanent cup disappears with wear, full length canine teeth may be present*
7 yrs	*intermediate incisor permanent cup disappears with wear, seven year hook on upper corner incisor, dental cup still visible on the corner incisor*
8 yrs	*corner incisor permanent cup disappears with wear, the first dental star appears on the central incisor, very beginnings of a dental star on the intermediate incisor*
9 yrs	*round central incisors with dental stars, intermediate incisors are becoming less oval and more round, corner incisors are oval, seven-year hook has disappeared*
10 yrs	*Galvayne's groove appears on the labial surface (facing the lips) of the upper corner incisor; central and intermediate incisors have become round at this point, central and intermediate incisors have dental stars in the middle of the teeth*
12 yrs	*all incisors are round, dental stars have waned to small yellow dots, Galvayne's groove has progressed one quarter of the way down the tooth*
15 yrs	*Galvayne's groove has progressed half-way down the upper corner incisor, the central incisor has become triangular in shape, round dental stars on all incisors*
20 yrs	*Galvayne's groove reaches the bottom of the tooth*

Source: Riegel and Hakola (1999).

Figure 1.3 Teeth.
Source: Rachel Monticelli-Turner.

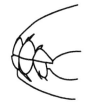

2 Years

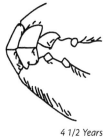

4 1/2 Years

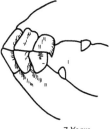

7 Years

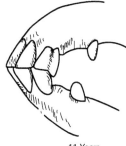

11 Years

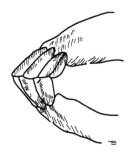

20 Years

NOTES:

Equine dentistry:

Because of the relative difference in the size of the upper jaw and lower jaw the horse tends to wear its teeth unevenly. As the upper jaw is wider this means the outside edge of the teeth experience less grinding activity. Therefore, they wear unevenly forming "points". The same happens on the inner edges of the lower teeth. These points can become sharp enough to cause discomfort (or even lacerations) on the horse's tongue and inner cheeks. Additionally horses can form hooks on the last molar, or can have an overgrown tooth if its opposing tooth is missing. All of these things can add up to less efficient chewing, discomfort, and biting issues. Therefore it is important to have a horse's teeth checked and possibly "floated" once or twice a year by a veterinarian or a qualified equine dental technician.

Figure 1.4 Grinding surfaces. *Source: Rachel Monticelli-Turner.*

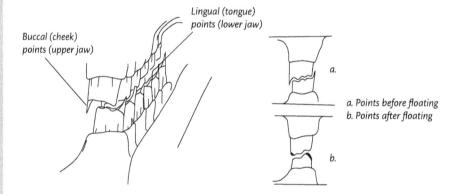

d.   *Tongue:* necessary for movement of feed from front to back of oral cavity; taste buds are located on its surface:

   i.   Very muscular; apex (rostral portion) body and root that attaches to hyoid apparatus and mandible; covered by keratinized stratified squamous epithelium (Frandson, Wilke, & Fails, 2009)

   ii.   Papillae: large projections, developed dorsally:

   1.   filiform—short and soft and give the tongue its velvety feel

   2.   fungiform*—interspersed in the filiform, mushroom-shaped

   3.   foliate*—resemble foliage; located on lateral margins near root of tongue

   4.   vallate*—found on caudal part of the tongue, arranged in a "V" shape; create the divide between the body and root of the tongue, shaped as large, circular projections, surrounded by a deep groove

   *contain taste buds

Figure 1.5 Dorsal view of the tongue and pharynx. *Source: Rachel Monticelli-Turner.*

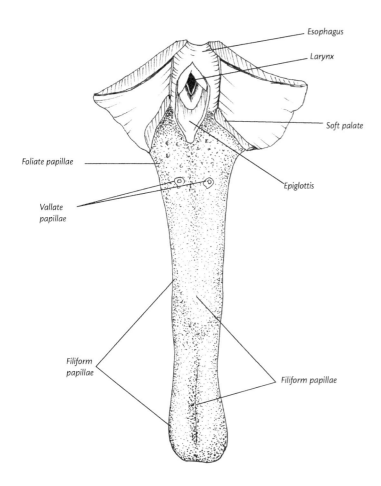

    e.   *Pharynx:* the common area for food and air; may include tonsils (groups of lymph nodules) A proper flow of food into the esophagus is accomplished by the action of the epiglottis covering the trachea during the act of swallowing.

2.   Esophagus

    a.   *Location:* extends from pharynx to stomach as a muscular tube (it lies dorsal to the trachea); passes through the mediastinum of the chest cavity and through the diaphragm at the area known as the esophageal hiatus

    b.   *Size:* 60″ in a mature horse; small and muscular

    c.   *Description:* contains a combination of skeletal and smooth types of muscle fibers

    d.   *Function:*

NOTES:

3. **Stomach**
   a. *Location:* caudal to left side of diaphragm
   b. *Size & shape:* relatively small in the horse, shaped like the letter "J" due to close proximity of cardia and pylorus regions
   c. *Function:*

   d. External stomach regions (Frandson, Wilke, & Fails, 2009) (*Label the underlined terms on Figure 1.6*):
      i. <u>Cardiac</u>: joined to esophagus, contains the well developed cardiac sphincter; this muscle makes it difficult for the horse to vomit
      ii. <u>Fundus</u>: large bulge near the cardia; enlarges into the saccus cecus
      iii. <u>Body</u>: allows for expansion
      iv. <u>Pylorus</u>: contains strong pyloric sphincter that regulates outflow of stomach contents
      v. <u>Greater curvature</u>: long, convex side
      vi. <u>Lesser curvature</u>: short, concave side

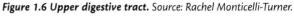

Figure 1.6 Upper digestive tract. *Source: Rachel Monticelli-Turner.*

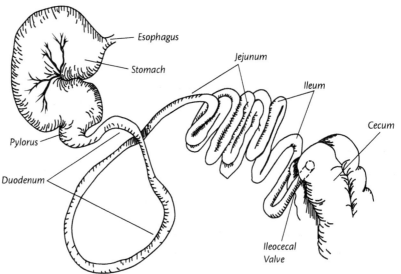

Comparative stomach sizes:

	Man	Pig	Horse	Cow
Body weight	75 kg	181 kg	454 kg	544 kg
	(165 lb)	(400 lb)	(1000 lb)	(1200 lb)
Total approx. stomach size	1 L	8 L	8 L	160 L
	(0.246 gal)	(1.97 gal)	(1.97 gal)	(39.36 gal)
	(1.057 qt)	(8.45 qt)	(8.45 qt)	(169.07 qt)

Source: Maynard and Loosli, 1975

Figure 1.7 Inside view of the stomach and cranial duodenum.
Source: Rachel Monticelli-Turner.

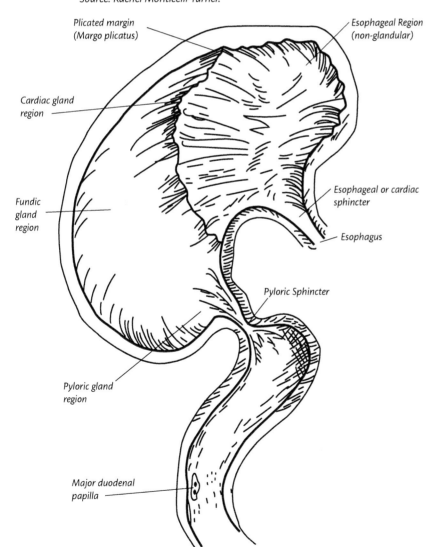

Plicated margin (Margo plicatus)

Esophageal Region (non-glandular)

Cardiac gland region

Fundic gland region

Esophageal or cardiac sphincter

Esophagus

Pyloric Sphincter

Pyloric gland region

Major duodenal papilla

NOTES:

Ulcers are much more common in horses than once thought. These can be brought on by stress (especially in foals and high-performance horses), certain medications (like nonsteroidal anti-inflammatories) plus other factors. The usual location for gastric ulcers would be near the plicated margin on the nonglandular side of the stomach.

e. Internal stomach regions:

   i.   *Nonglandular:* the esophageal region is the expanded portion of external cardiac region

   ii. *Margo plicatus:* the demarcation between nonglandular and glandular internal regions

   iii. *Glandular:* made up of three internal regions (see chart below); interspersed with enteroendocrine cells (these secrete hormones which affect secretory and muscular activity of the digestive tract)

Cardiac gland	mucus	protects stomach lining; small in the horse
Fundic gland	pepsin	acts on proteins; largest glandular area in the horse
Pyloric gland	mucus	protection of stomach lining

4. **Small intestine (refer to Figures 1.6 and 1.8)**

   a. *Location:* attaches to pyloric region of stomach

   b. *Size:* length in mature horse is approximately 70′; 12 gallon or 45 liter capacity

   c. *Functions:*

   d. *Regions* (locate each underlined region on Figure 1.6):

      i.   <u>Duodenum</u>: first part, 3 ft, receives secretions from liver and pancreas

      ii. <u>Jejunum</u>: middle part and longest portion—54 ft; longer supporting mesentery

      iii. <u>Ileum</u>: last part; 10–12 ft; connects to cecum in horse at *ileo-cecal junction*

B. *Primary organs of digestion: The lower digestive tract*

Complete the outline below while studying the unique features of the primary organs that make up the lower digestive tract of the horse. Locate all organs on Figures 1.8 and 1.9.

1. **Cecum**

   a. *Location:* the base of the cecum (location for the ileo-cecal junction) is closest to the horse's right hip, it then extends ventrally and cranially (toward the diaphragm) to the apex as a "blind sac"; the exit for cecal ingesta takes place from the cecal-colic junction located near the ileo-cecal junction.

   b. *Size:* In the mature horse, the cecum may contain 8 gallons (about 33 liters) of watery, fibrous ingesta and extends approximately 4 feet within the horse's abdomen.

The cecum of a horse (which is a major site of microbial digestion) is equivalent to the appendix in a human (which is of questionable use).

Figure 1.8 Organs of the equine digestive system.
Source: Carmel Keeley.

1. Oral Cavity
2. Pharynx
3. Esophagus
4. Trachea
5. Stomach
6. Pancreas
7. Liver
8. Duodenum

9. Jejunum
10. Ileum
11. Base of Cecum
12. Body of Cecum
13. Apex of Cecum
14. Ceco-colic Fold
15. Right Ventral Colon
16. Sternal Flexure

17. Left Ventral Colon
18. Pelvic Flexure
19. Left Dorsal Colon
20. Diaphragmatic Flexure
21. Right Dorsal Colon
22. Transverse Colon
23. Small Colon
24. Rectum

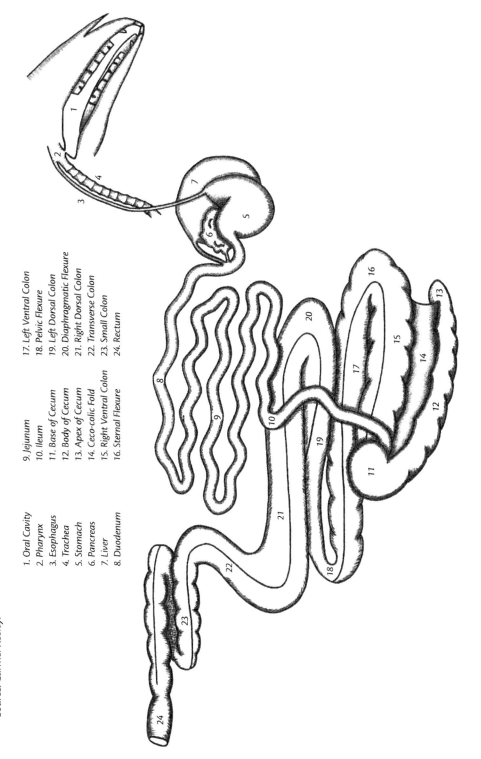

NOTES:

Impaction colic is more likely to occur in places where there is a narrowing or turning of the gut pathway. Therefore common places for impactions are at the diaphragmatic and sternal flexures of the large colon (turns), and especially the pelvic flexure (a narrowing and an upwards turn against gravity).

c. *Functions:*

d. *Unique features/appearance:* The large size and function of the horse's cecum makes it unique among animals of its size; other animals with similar digestive properties include the rabbit, the elephant, and the rhinoceros.

2. **Large colon**

a. *Location:* It begins at the ceco-colic junction near the base of the cecum and ends with the transverse colon, making three turns throughout the horse's abdomen.

b. *Size:* In the mature horse, the large colon may contain up to 16 gallons of ingesta (60 liters) and, when stretched out, may cover 12 feet.

c. *Functions:*

d. *Unique features/appearance:* The large size and capacity and the narrowing of the organ at each flexure makes feeding consistency and frequency along with proper hydration of the horse critical to avoid such issues as colic.

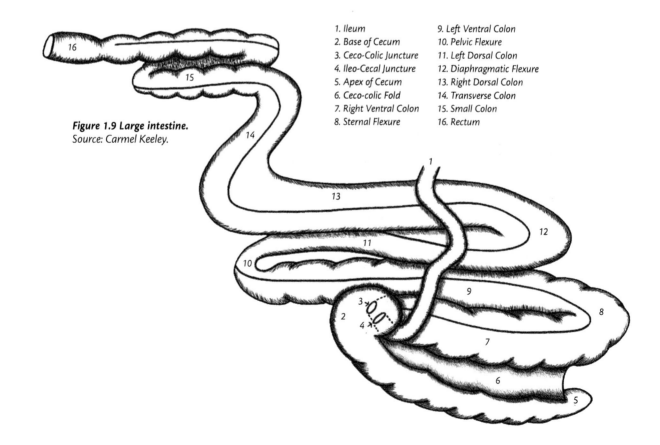

Figure 1.9 Large intestine.
Source: Carmel Keeley.

1. Ileum
2. Base of Cecum
3. Ceco-Colic Juncture
4. Ileo-Cecal Juncture
5. Apex of Cecum
6. Ceco-colic Fold
7. Right Ventral Colon
8. Sternal Flexure
9. Left Ventral Colon
10. Pelvic Flexure
11. Left Dorsal Colon
12. Diaphragmatic Flexure
13. Right Dorsal Colon
14. Transverse Colon
15. Small Colon
16. Rectum

Figure 1.10 Position of organs of digestion, right view. *Source: Rachel Monticelli-Turner.*

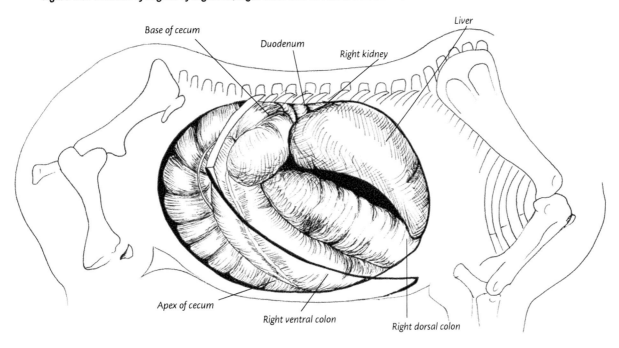

Figure 1.11 Position of organs of digestion, left view. *Source: Rachel Monticelli-Turner.*

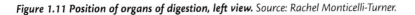
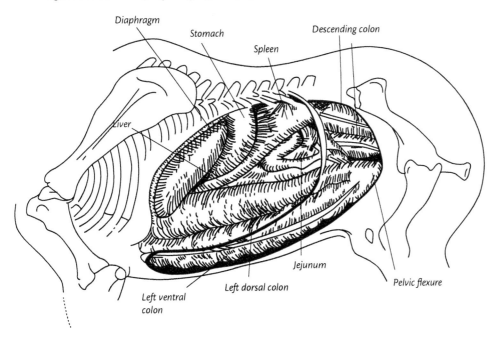

The cecum, large colon, and small colon (which includes the transverse colon) are also collectively referred to as the large intestine of the horse.

   e. *Regions and flexures*—in sequence from cecum to small colon:
       i.   Right ventral colon
       ii.   Sternal flexure
       iii. Left ventral colon
       iv.   Pelvic flexure
       v.   Left dorsal colon
       vi.   Diaphragmatic flexure
       vii. Right dorsal colon

3. **Small colon**
   a. *Location:* begins with the transverse colon at the end of the right dorsal colon (where it crosses the horse's midline just cranial to the root of the greater mesentery) and ends with the descending portion that joins to the rectum.

   b. *Size:* holds approximately 3–4 gallons or 11–15 liters of ingesta and extends 10–12 feet.

   c. *Functions:*

   d. *Appearance:* larger in diameter than the small intestine; internally, the contents are drier than the large colon contents.

4. **Rectum and anus**
   a. *Location:* the rectum begins at the pelvic inlet and ends at the exterior opening of the digestive tract, called the anus.

   b. *Size:* the rectum is generally about 1 foot long and lies dorsal to numerous organs.

   c. *Functions:*

   d. *Unique features:* due to its position, rectal palpation is important in enabling the diagnosis of certain disorders, such as colic; or in determining the reproductive status of mares.

C. Secondary organs of digestion

The salivary glands, the pancreas, and the liver all provide secretions that aid in the process of digestion, but since feed does not pass through any of them, they are all considered to be secondary organs of digestion (Frandson, Wilke, & Fails, 2009).

1. **Salivary glands**
   a. Parotid glands:
      i. *Location:* ventral to the ear in relation to caudal border of the mandible
      ii. *Secretions:* serous (watery) saliva
   b. Mandibular glands:
      i. *Location:* ventral to parotid glands and caudal to mandible
      ii. *Secretions:* mucus (protective) and serous saliva (mixed glands)
   c. Sublingual glands:
      i. *Location:* central to the tongue near floor of the mouth
      ii. *Secretions:* mixed (mucus and serous)

2. **Pancreas**
   a. *Location:* A small lobe-like organ, the pancreas lies next to the first part of the duodenum and adjacent to the stomach.
   b. *Secretions and functions:*
      i. Exocrine: produces sodium bicarbonate and digestive enzymes that empty into the proximal duodenum
      ii. Endocrine: produces the hormones insulin and glucagon that assist with blood sugar regulation

3. **Liver**
   a. *Location:* This large organ lies just caudal to the diaphragm and consists of several lobes.
   b. *Digestive secretions and functions:* This includes bile that moves directly from the liver to the proximal duodenum and is involved with the break-down of fats. The liver is a major detoxifying organ and venous blood leaving the digestive system travels through the liver for filtration before it passes back through the heart and lungs.

NOTES:

Unlike humans, horses do not have a gallbladder! The gallbladder's function in other animals is to store bile from the liver and secrete it when there is fat to be digested in the small intestine. The horse, however, secretes small amounts of bile constantly, and hence doesn't need a storage area. Some other animals that lack gallbladders are elephants, rats, and rhinoceroses.

Table 1.1 Enzymes in Digestion

Location	Product/ Enzyme secreted	Acts on?	End result?
Mouth	Ptyalin	starch	maltose
	Salivary amylase	amylase	maltose
Stomach	HCl	dissolves minerals	
	Pepsinogen (+ HCl = pepsin)	proteins	amino acids
	Rennin	milk	coagulated milk
Small Intestine	Peptidase	proteins	amino acids
	Maltase	maltose (simple sugars)	glucose
	Sucrase	sucrose (simple sugars)	glucose
	Lactase	lactose (simple sugars)	glucose
	Enterokinase	trypsinogen enzyme from pancreas	activated trypsin enzyme
Pancreas	Trypsin (activated by enterokinase from small intestine) Chemotrypsin	proteins	amino acids
	Pancreatic amylase	starches	oligosaccharides (these are further digested by maltase and sucrase to monosaccharides)
	Pancreatic lipase	fats	fatty acids and monoglycerides
	Sodium bicarbonate	chyme (from stomach)	raises the pH and enhances the effects of pancreatic enzymes
	Insulin	glucose	causes glucose uptake by tissues and organs
	Glucagon	glycogen	causes break-down of glycogen to glucose in the liver (glycogenolysis)
		fatty acids & proteins	production of glucose from non-carbohydrate sources in the liver and kidneys (gluconeogenesis)
Liver	Bile	fats	emulsifies globules
Large intestine	Only microbial digestion!	fiber, mostly	Volatile fatty Acids and microbial protein
All over	Mucus	protects gut lining	protects gut lining

For additional information:

Oke, Stacey DVM, MSc (2018, July). Journey through the Equine GI Tract. The Horse. Retrieved from http://thehorse.com/159348/journey-through-the-equine-gi-tract/.

YouTube videos:

The equine digestive system:
https://www.youtube.com/watch?v=tuzTJ77IQAY

The horse's digestive system:
youtube.com/watch?v=81qk7igz9L4

3D horse digestion guide:
youtube.com/watch?v=maWXVKI-gq4

References:

Frandson, R., Wilke, W., & Fails, A. (2009). *Anatomy and Physiology of Farm Animals.* (7th ed.). Philadelphia, PA: Lippincott, Williams and Wilkins.

Maynard, L., & Loosli, J. (1975). *Animal Nutrition.* 6th edition. New York: McGraw-Hill Book Company.

Pence, P. (2002). *Equine Dentistry A Practical Guide.* Philadelphia, PA: Lippincott, Williams and Wilkins.

Riegel, R., & Hakola, S. (1999). *Illustrated Atlas of Clinical Equine Anatomy and Common Disorders of the Horse* (Vol. 2). Marysville, OH: Equistar Publications, Ltd.

Supplemental Activity
STRINGING IT ALL TOGETHER

Materials:

- String
- Scissors
- Tape measure

- Tape or labels that can be written on
- Lengths of all the primary organs of digestion
- Spool to wrap finished product around

Objective:

The idea is to have students gain a better understanding of the true length of the equine digestive tract by measuring out the lengths of the primary digestive organs and marking them on string.

Activity:

1. Add all the lengths of the primary digestive organs and make sure you have at least that length of string.

2. Fasten the string to the spool.

3. Measure one rectum length of string from the spool. (We start at this end so that the beginning of the digestive tract will be on the outside when the string is wound on the spool.)

4. Mark the string by folding a length of tape or a label over the string and sticking it back to itself. Write "rectum" on the tape or label and indicate its length.

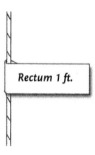

5. Continue this process working backwards marking the rest of the primary digestive organs.

6. Use the scissors to trim off excess string.

7. Stretch out your finished product with a friend to get an idea of the true length of the equine digestive tract. Wind your string onto your spool for safekeeping.

8. If you are super ambitious, repeat the process for the human digestive system. Compare the lengths of the two digestive tracts. Can you think of any reasons for the difference in length?

Name_____

Lab Section_____

Lab 1 Assignment
THE EQUINE DIGESTIVE SYSTEM

1. Observe specimens and diagrams related to the equine digestive tract, making note of their unique features, shapes, and sizes. Then complete the chart below:

Organ	Location	Size/Shape	Function(s)
a. lips			
b. tongue			
c. teeth			
d. pharynx			
e. esophagus			
f. stomach			
g. small intestine			
h. cecum			
i. large colon			
j. small colon			
k. rectum			

2. The location of nutrient digestion in the horse is an important factor in successful feeding. Research and list which digestive organ or organs are involved with the digestion and absorption of each nutrient listed. If an accessory organ is involved, please include that along with the primary digestive organ that is associated with it.

	Location of Digestion	*Location of Absorption*
a. carbohydratessimple sugars		
complex carbohydrates (fiber)		
b. proteins		
c. lipids		
d. minerals		
e. vitamins		
f. water		

3. The goal of a horse owner is to maximize digestion and absorption of feed nutrients. How might the following factors impact both digestion and absorption?

   a. The quantity of feed intake at a single feeding.

   b. The order of providing feeds (hay versus grain versus water).

   c. The processing of feeds (such as crimping, grinding, or steaming).

4. Describe (do not just list) three basic differences between the equine digestive tract and the ruminant digestive tract.

5. You recently inherited a small Cleveland Bay breeding farm from an obscure relative that passed away. Unfortunately, because your new Cleveland Bays have no markings and all other physical characteristics are similar because they are all related, your obscure relative was the only one able to tell them apart. Luckily you found a folder with papers on all the current horses. Use your knowledge of teeth and aging along with the descriptions on the next page to determine which horse is which in this brood mare paddock.

   a. Little Red: age 2.5
   b. Big Red: age 5
   c. Little Red Riding Hood: age 11
   d. Maroon: age 15
   e. Rojo: age 25

Horse descriptions:

Horse 1: This horse has what is known as a "full mouth," or full dentition. All of the incisors have cups and the canines are fully erupted, though they are small.

Horse 2: Galvayne's groove has made an appearance. The central and intermediate incisors have a rounded appearance. The corner incisors are moving from oval to round in their shape. The dental stars are waning.

Horse 3: The central permanent incisor is beginning to erupt. There are no wolf teeth. Second permanent premolar has erupted.

Horse 4: Galvayne's groove is half-way down the upper corner incisor. The central incisor has become triangular in shape. There are round dental stars on all of the incisors.

Horse 5: All of the incisors are triangular. Galvayne's groove is half-way down the upper corner incisor. The teeth are more slanted than the #4 horse.

Laboratory 2
PLANT IDENTIFICATION

Source: Rachel Monticelli-Turner.

Introduction:

As covered and illustrated in Laboratory 1, the horse is designed to eat a diet based on plant material. Plants have the potential to be both nutritious and non-nutritious. A horse owner or stable manager should have a thorough knowledge of the plants that grow in his or her area, including those that provide nutritional value and those that are not nutritious or that are not safe for horses to consume.

Objectives:

When finished with the material from this laboratory, the student should be able to:

1. Provide a definition for both nutritious and non-nutritious plants.
2. In the category of nutritious plants:
    a. Describe four characteristics of all grasses.
    b. Describe four characteristics of all legumes.
3. In the category of non-nutritious plants:
    a. Identify two to four nuisance types of vegetation in one's geographic area.
    b. Identify two to four plants in one's geographic area that are poisonous or harmful to horses.

Questions for further discussion:

1. When is it appropriate to feed grass forage to horses?
2. When is it appropriate to feed legume forage to horses?
3. What are some of the more common misconceptions regarding grasses and legumes?
4. What harmful or poisonous plant located in your area was the most surprising to you?

Manual of Equine Nutrition and Feeding Management, First Edition.
Carol Z. Buckhout and Barbara E. Lindberg.
© 2022 John Wiley & Sons, Inc. Published 2022 by John Wiley & Sons, Inc.
Companion website: www.wiley.com/go/buckhout/manual

NOTES:

Some common grasses:
(not all grow well in every
climate zone!)
Timothy

Orchard grass

Smooth brome grass

Bluestem

Bluegrass

Reed canary grass

Rye grass

Bermuda grass

Bahia

Oats (as hay or as straw + grain)

Wheat (as hay or as straw + grain)

Barley (as hay or as straw + grain)

Some common legumes:

Alfalfa

Common (Dutch) clover

Ladino clover

Alsike clover

Red clover

Birdsfoot trefoil

Nitrogen fixation:

**Nitrogen fixation involves
the process by which gaseous
nitrogen can be extracted
from the environment and
added to the soil via bacteria
that can be found in the
roots of certain plants, such
as legumes.**

Nutritious Plants:

Plants that provide useful feeding value in the form of nutrients to the animals that consume them are considered to be nutritious. Forages, a category of nutritious plants, may be classified as follows (Lewis, 1996):

A. Grasses

1. Plant characteristics:
   a. *Height:* tall, thin stalk; may reach 24–36″ at maturity
   b. *Leaf content:* a few flat leaves grouped at the bottom of the plant
   c. *Maturity:* a group of seeds, called the "head" appear at the top and become larger with age; the joints of the stem lighten with age
   d. *Color:* light green when immature; this changes to a range of gold to brown as the plant matures and the indigestible lignin content increases
   e. *Growth rate:* the cool, wet weather of northern spring climates is ideal for growing grasses such as orchard grass, timothy, Kentucky bluegrass, and brome grass; they dominate the fields by late May.
2. Uses:
   a. *Stems and leaves:* popular for pastures and may provide nutritious forage for hay when harvested at the appropriate time; may also be used for bedding (straw) if the source is a cereal grain
   b. *Seed portion:* contains concentrated nutrients, such as energy and some may be used as grains.

B. Legumes

1. Plant characteristics include:
   a. *Height:* short, branched stalk; may reach 18–24″ at maturity
   b. *Leaf content:* numerous leaves
   c. *Maturity:* a characteristic flower appears
   d. *Color:* dark green throughout their growth period
   e. *Growth rate:* slower than grasses because they prefer warmer temperatures
   f. Nitrogen fixation properties (due to bacteria in root nodules) contribute to their characteristic dark green color and nutritious properties
   g. Excellent source of nutrients, including protein, energy, and calcium; may be too nutritious for some horses.

2. Uses:

    a. *Stems and leaves:* used for pasture or hay; also processed products such as alfalfa cubes and pellets

    b. *Seed portion:* some legumes provide concentrates, such as soybeans

    Additional information related to forages will be covered in Labs 3 and 4.

Study the diagrams of grasses and legumes provided on the next pages. Compare the diagrams with the specimens provided in the laboratory. Make notes of the distinct differences and similarities between the various plants.

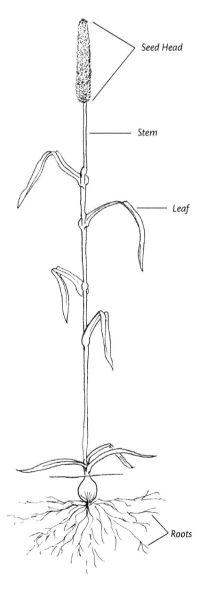

Seed Head

Stem

Leaf

Roots

Figure 2.1 Timothy grass: *Phleum pratense.*
Source: Rachel Monticelli-Turner.

NOTES:

Cool vs. warm season grasses

These plants define themselves. Those that prefer to grow in temperatures that range between 60–75 degrees F are labeled as cool season grasses while warm season grasses prefer temperatures between 85 and 90 degrees F. Cool season grasses such as timothy, orchard grass, and Kentucky bluegrass store their energy as fructan, a polysaccharide, which is not digested in the small intestine of the horse. Excessive levels of fructan in a horse's diet can create digestive imbalances in the hind gut leading to undesirable situations such as colic and laminitis. Since strong sunlight draws the fructan content of grasses up into their stems, diet management of horses consuming cool season grasses may include grazing in the early morning hours or using grazing muzzles to limit the amount of grass intake. Stress on cool season grasses, such as over grazing, can cause fructans to concentrate in the lower portion of the stems, also resulting in laminitis on the unsuspecting grazing horse.

NOTES:

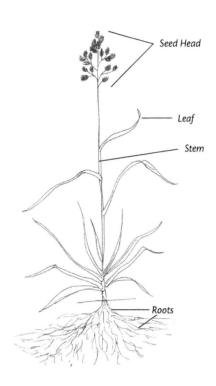

Figure 2.2 Orchard grass: *Dactylis glomerata*.
Source: Rachel Monticelli-Turner.

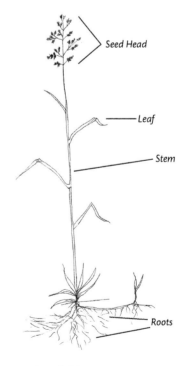

Figure 2.3 Canada bluegrass: *Poa compressa*.
Source: Rachel Monticelli-Turner.

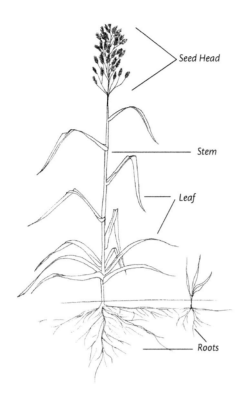

Seed Head

Stem

Leaf

Roots

Figure 2.4 Smooth brome grass: *Bromus inermis.*
Source: Rachel Monticelli-Turner.

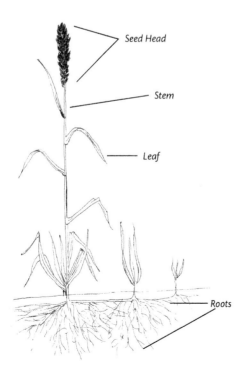

Seed Head

Stem

Leaf

Roots

Figure 2.5 Reed canary grass: *Phalaris arundinacea.*
Source: Rachel Monticelli-Turner.

NOTES:

Please note that when identifying forages, Figures 2.6 and 2.7 are not drawn to the same scale.

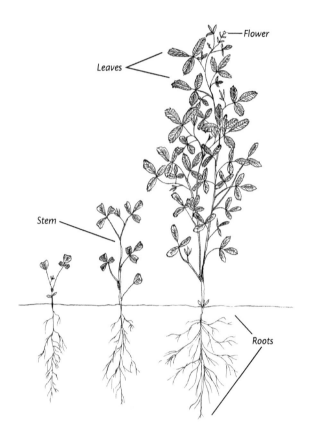

Figure 2.6 Alfalfa: *Medicago sativa*. *Source: Rachel Monticelli-Turner.*

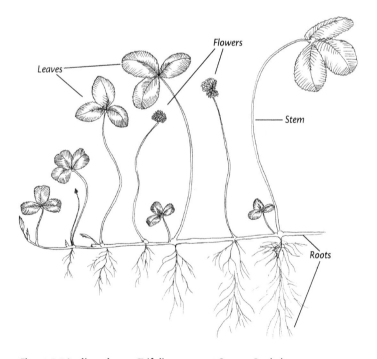

Figure 2.7 Ladino clover: *Trifolium repens*. *Source: Rachel Monticelli-Turner.*

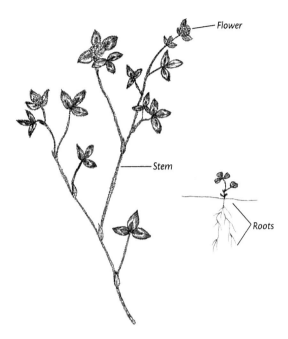

Figure 2.8 Red clover: *Trifolium pratense.* Source: Rachel Monticelli-Turner.

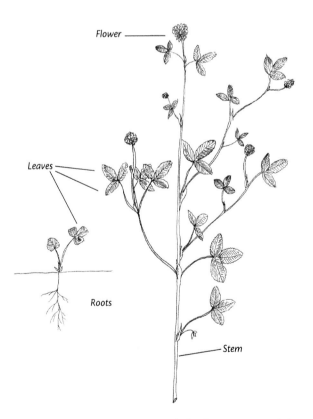

Figure 2.9 Alsike clover: *Trifolium hybridium.* Source: Rachel Monticelli-Turner.

NOTES:

NOTES:

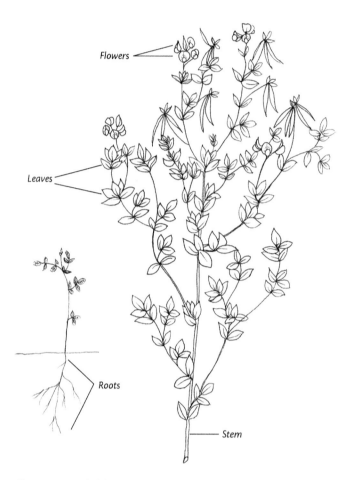

*Figure 2.10   **Birdsfoot trefoil:** **Lotus tenuis.** Source: Rachel Monticelli-Turner.*

Non-Nutritious Plants:

These plants provide little or no feeding value to animals that consume them. They may be poisonous or harmful to a horse.

A. *Nuisance plants: these are not poisonous to the horse, but they do not supply proper nutritional value*

1.   Weeds—anything that is not intended to be present in an area where horses are grazing or in forage that is harvested for horse feeding (ex: crab grass).

2.   They may inhibit other plants from growing (ex: dandelion).

3.   They may cause skin or eye irritations (ex: nettles, burdocks).

B. *Feed and bedding conditions that are harmful to horses*

Using information provided by the instructor and consulting the references at the end of this section, list symptoms characteristic of the different types of poisoning or health risks. State the conditions that can cause the situation.

1. Plants affected by fungi
    a. Corn (moldy corn disease)

    b. Sweet clover

    c. Fescue

2. Contaminants in forage and bedding
    a. Botulism

    b. Blister beetles

    c. Trash and foreign objects

3. Bedding
    a. Black walnut shavings

    b. Straw baled wet and/or dusty straw

Mold can happen if storage conditions are not ideal. Feed that has become wet or that was baled wet has a greater risk of becoming moldy. Older feed is also at risk, be sure to know how long the feed has been stored.

C. Poisonous plants: These will cause some sort of external or internal damage to the horse, affecting its health and, in some cases, even causing death

1. The species will vary, depending on climate (temperature and moisture), soil conditions, and geographic region.

2. Some are poisonous when fresh, others are more potent when dried.

3. **Horses usually will not eat poisonous plants if there is enough *nutritious* forage to eat (Knight, 1996).**

Using information provided by the instructor and consulting the references at the end of this section, list symptoms of the different types of poisoning or health risks. State the conditions that can cause the situation.

1. Plants causing photosensitization (white areas on a horse look sunburned)
    a. St. John's wort

    b. Alsike clover

2. Trees can be dangerous especially if a tree or a cut branch falls in a pasture. Horses are curious, and they investigate by eating.
    a. Red maple

    b. Oak

3. Ornamental plants
    a. Yew

    b. Rhododendron and mountain laurels

    c. Oleander

4. Sudden-death inducing plants
    a. Poison hemlock and water hemlock

    b. Johnson grass and sudan grass

5. Selenium excess
    a. Causes

    b. Obligate selenium accumulator plants

    c. Secondary selenium accumulator plants

NOTES:

NOTES:

6. Other common plants and their effects
    a. Bracken fern

    b. Buttercups

    c. Choke cherry

    d. Horse chestnut and buckeye

    e. Horsetail

    f. Milkweed

    g. Nightshade plants: jimson weed, potato, and tomato

AVOID PLANT POISONING BY FEEDING GOOD-QUALITY HAY OR
PASTURE, CLEAN WATER AND SALT. MAINTAIN FENCES AND PREVENT BOREDOM!

For additional information:

Equus Magazine. (2007, July: Updated 2017, March). A guide to common poisonous plants. 59. Retrieved from http://www.equisearch.com/articles/common-poisonous-plants-chart-8311/.

Equus Magazine. (2004, June). 10 most poisonous plants for horses. *Equus*. Retrieved from http://www.equisearch.com/horses_care/nutrition/feeds/poisonousplants_041105/.

Helpful websites/links on toxic plants:

Colorado State University:
http://www.csuvth.colostate.edu/poisonous_plants/

University of New Hampshire:
https://extension.unh.edu/sites/default/files/migrated_unmanaged_files/Resource000623_Rep645.pdf

References:

Knight, A. (1996). Plant Poisoning of Horses. In L. Lewis, *Feeding and Care of the Horse* (2nd ed.). pp. 300–345. Media, PA: Lippincott, Williams and Wilkins.

Lewis, L. (1996). *Feeding and Care of the Horse* (2nd ed.). Media, PA: Lippincott, Williams and Wilkens.

Laboratory 2
ACTIVITIES

1. Observe the various plants that are either provided in class by the instructor or starting with Figure 2.1 of this lab. Be certain to identify whether they are classified as grasses or legumes and be able to list their individual identifying characteristics.

2. Complete the lab section about harmful and poisonous plants. List plants found in your area that are considered to be either harmful or poisonous. Use sources listed in the "For additional information," "Helpful websites," and "Reference" sections to answer this question.

Supplemental Activity
PASTURE WALK MANUAL

Materials:

- Pictures or samples of harmful plants
- Local resources on harmful plants

Objective:

The idea is to have students create a tool that will be useful in identifying plants harmful to horses.

Activity:

1. Compile a list of plants harmful to horses in your area. (The plants listed in this manual are a good starting point, but modify your list according to your area.)

2. Find pictures and/or samples of the plants you have chosen.

3. Create a manual that local stable owners could use while checking their pastures and hay for harmful plants. You many use the template on the following page or create your own format.

4. Search a pasture for harmful plants using your manual.

Place samples and/or pictures here

Name of Plant: _____

Toxic parts:	Symptoms of poisoning:
Time of year toxic:	Treatment:
Conditions it grows well in:	Other considerations:

Name_____

Lab Section_____

Equine Nutrition Lab 2 Assignment
NUTRITIOUS AND NON-NUTRITIOUS PLANTS FOR HORSES

1. To reinforce the difference between grasses and legumes, complete the table below, listing four (4) physical characteristics that are unique to each type of plant and providing three (3) specific examples of each type. Also, suggest categories of horses (maintenance, growing, breeding, idle, or working), not specific breeds of horses, that would be most appropriate, in your opinion, to feed each type of forage.

	Physical Characteristics	Plant Examples	Horse categories
Grass:	1.	1.	1.
	2.	2.	2.
	3.	3.	
	4.		
Legume:	1.	1.	1.
	2.	2.	2.
	3.	3.	
	4.		

2.   Research a minimum of four (4) harmful or poisonous plants found in your home geographic area. Fill out the next four (4) pages with the information that you find.

Place samples and/or pictures here

Name of plant: _____

Toxic parts:	Symptoms of poisoning:
Time of year toxic:	**Treatment:**
Conditions it grows well in:	**Other considerations:**

Place samples and/or pictures here

Name of plant: _____

Toxic parts:	Symptoms of poisoning:
Time of year toxic:	Treatment:
Conditions it grows well in:	Other considerations:

Place samples and/or pictures here

Name of plant: _____

Toxic parts:	Symptoms of poisoning:
Time of year toxic:	**Treatment:**
Conditions it grows well in:	**Other considerations:**

Place samples and/or pictures here

Name of plant: _____

Toxic parts:	Symptoms of poisoning:
Time of year toxic:	Treatment:
Conditions it grows well in:	Other considerations:

Laboratory 3
FORAGE 1: PASTURE

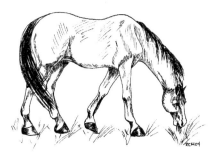

Source: Rachel Monticelli-Turner.

Introduction:

Laboratories 1 and 2 have provided proof that nutritious forages are the foundation of a horse's diet. Pastures are a popular venue for the general health and well being of the horse. Laboratory 3 will review and further explore the properties of forages and apply their use to pastures. Topics included are: types of pastures, advantages and disadvantages of pastures, varieties of forages that provide quality pastures and challenges of pasture management.

Objectives:

When finished with the material from this laboratory, the student should be able to:

1. List four characteristics of forages.
2. Discuss three functions of forages for the digestive system.
3. Review classifications of forages.
4. Define the term "quality" in regards to forages.
5. Define the term "pasture".
6. Describe three types of pastures that may be used for horses.
7. Discuss five advantages and five disadvantages of pastures.
8. Suggest five important pasture management practices.
9. Determine the optimum number of horses per acre of pasture, based on its location and forage quality.
10. Identify non-nutritious plants that may be found in pastures in your geographic area.

Questions for further discussion:

1. What are the most abundant pasture plants found in your specific area?
2. How would you re-organize your own permanent pasture into a rotational situation?
3. Suggest a combination of grasses and legumes that would be acceptable in a pasture mix.

Manual of Equine Nutrition and Feeding Management, First Edition.
Carol Z. Buckhout and Barbara E. Lindberg.
© 2022 John Wiley & Sons, Inc. Published 2022 by John Wiley & Sons, Inc.
Companion website: www.wiley.com/go/buckhout/manual

*Mcal or "megacalorie"
is equal to 1000 kilocal-
ories (Kcal) or 1,000,000
calories (c).*

*Digestible energy (DE):
measured in megacalo-
ries (Mcal), the digestible
energy of a feed is the
amount of energy digested
and absorbed by a horse.
Determined by subtract-
ing fecal energy from gross
energy, DE is greatly affected
by the amounts and types
of fibrous components of a
plant. Plants with higher CF,
ADF, or NDF (and lignin)
values will have lower
DE values.*

Gross Energy − Fecal Energy = DE

*Crude fiber (CF) is an
estimate of the cell wall
contents of a plant. However
it does not accurately represent the plant's hemicellulose
or the lignin content, and
therefore is not the most
accurate measure of plant
fiber. However, crude fiber
continues to be a common
value used with horse
rations today.*

General overview:

As a nonruminant herbivore, the horse requires nutritious plant material, or forage, each day to provide nutrients and fiber. Pasture can be a source of nutritious forages. It also can be important to the psychological health of a horse.

Forage facts

Forage refers to the portion of the horse's diet that provides high quantities of fiber. The nutritional value (or quality) of the fiber can be affected by numerous factors including the actual type of forage as well as the growing, harvesting, and storage conditions. The outline below provides some basic facts about forages.

A. General characteristics of forages:
1. Vegetative (leaves and stems)
2. High in fiber content and low in digestible energy:
    a. Crude fiber (CF) generally between 28–38%
    b. Digestible energy (DE) usually 0.9–1.1 Mcal/lb or 1.9–2.4 Mcal/kg
3. Can be sources of energy, protein, vitamins, and minerals
4. Relatively inexpensive to feed

B. Functions of forages:
1. Stimulation of the gastrointestinal tract due to the relatively high fiber content
2. Provide a source of important nutrients, depending on the plant types involved
3. Essential to cecal and large colon microbial growth and function

C. Classification (review information from Laboratory 2):
1. Legumes
    a. excellent source of energy, protein, Vitamin A, and minerals (calcium, phosphorus, magnesium)
    b. high crude protein content is due to nitrogen fixation properties and can approach 20% (NRC, 2007)
2. Grasses
    a. lower nutrient content than legumes
    b. with no nitrogen fixation and less leaf material, crude protein content can be much lower than legumes (NRC, 2007)
    c. they can meet the nutrient needs of maintenance horses and possibly those exercised at a light activity level

D. Forage quality:
  1. Refers to the nutrient content of a specific forage
  2. Factors affecting quality
    a. soil type
    b. growing conditions (wet/dry)
    c. harvesting date and conditions
    d. storage method and length of storage time
    e. plant species

E. Forage utilization:
  1. Pastures: fresh forage; the most natural form of forage for horses
  2. Hay: dried forage
    a. traditional bales (various sizes)
    b. processed into hay cubes or pellets
    c. processed, short chop provided in bags
  3. Greenchop: freshly chopped forage; fed most frequently to dairy or beef cattle
  4. Silage: fermented forage (as a method to preserve large quantities of forage) fed mostly to dairy or beef cattle

Pastures for horses

A. Definition: An area of land with forage so that animals may graze; almost half of the continental United States is covered by pasture or range land (Lewis, 1996).

B. Types of pastures:
  1. Permanent
    a. last for many years
    b. commonly found in areas not used for other purposes
    c. include hillsides, lowlands, and non-cropable lands
  2. Semi-permanent or rotational
    a. usually 2 to 7 years between reseedings
    b. may be used as part of an established crop rotation
    c. may be very efficient in maximizing the grazing potential of an area of land
  3. Temporary or supplemental
    a. used for short periods for supplemental grazing
    b. often used when other forms of pasture are non-productive
    c. often seeded with annual grasses (as opposed to perennials)

Acid Detergent Fiber (ADF) more accurately represents the fiber value of a plant as it includes most of the plant's cellulose and lignin content. Higher ADF values indicate lower feed digestibility. ADF does not accurately include the plant hemicellulose content, which is efficiently utilized by the horse.

Neutral Detergent Fiber (NDF) is the most accurate measure of the components of the plant cell wall, including cellulose (nearly all of it), hemicellulose (over 50% of it), and lignin. It is the best estimation of forage quality. Higher NDF levels of a plant generally indicate lower dry matter intakes and lower nutrient content.

Lignin is an indigestible plant cell wall component that increases with plant maturity. The higher the lignin content, the lower the digestibility of the plant. This proves the importance of feeding quality forages.

NOTES:

C. Advantages of pastures
    1. They lessen feed costs.
    2. They lessen hazards of nutritional deficiencies.
    3. They reduce the threat of communicable diseases.
    4. They require less capital for buildings and equipment.
    5. They require lower level of management skills.
    6. They may improve soil conservation.
    7. They provide exercise in addition to grazing opportunities.
    8. They are a good use of land not suited to crop production.
    9. They provide needed "down time" for confined animals and may enhance conception rates in mares.
    10. Other.

D. Disadvantages of pasture
    1. The land may be more productive when used for crops.
    2. Some areas require large amounts of land to support one animal.
    3. Poor soil will create lower quality plants.
    4. They require maintenance and proper management.
    5. Horses may be prone to laminitis due to lush pasture forage.
    6. They may contain harmful and toxic plants.
    7. Forage losses may occur due to trampling, urination, and manure.
    8. The forage may reach maturity too soon for it all to be nutritious.
    9. Insects and rodents may live and breed in some pastures.
    10. Other.

E. Pasture plants: (other pasture plants may be grown according to location and climatic conditions)
    1. Nutritious examples
        a. bluegrass
        b. clover
        c. timothy
        d. alfalfa
        e. other:
    2. Non-nutritious or poisonous examples
        a. dandelion
        b. buttercups
        c. burdocks
        d. milkweed
        e. other:

F. Horse numbers per acre of pasture: This changes according to the growing season. For example, in May and June when the moisture content of the soil enhances plant growth, the acres of pasture needed to support one horse in the northeast ranges from 0.5 to 1. However, in late July and August when the growing rate of forage is dramatically reduced, the number of acres required to support one horse can range from 1 to 3.5.

This is also influenced by the type of forage plants found in the pasture (Chamberlain, et. al. 2004).

1. Forage quantity and quality determines its grazing value.

2. Eastern U.S.: with seasonal pastures, 1 acre per horse is the minimum recommendation for grazing value for a time period of 8–12 hours per day (Chamberlain, et. al. 2004).

3. Western U.S.: with less potential of grazing value, several acres (to much more than this) per horse is recommended.

4. One acre = 43,560 square feet; knowing pasture dimensions will help to determine acreage and potential load rate of the pasture.

References:

Chamberlain, E., Foulk, D., Margentino, M., Mickel, B., & Westendorf, M. (2004). *Agricultural management practices for commercial equine operations.* Bulletin E296. Retrieved from Rutgers University New Jersey Agricultural Experiment Station website: https://esc.rutgers.edu/wp-content/uploads/2014/11/Agricultural-Management-Practices-for-Commercial-Equine-Operations.pdf..

Lewis, L. (1996). *Feeding and Care of the Horse* (2nd ed.) Media, PA: Lippincott, Williams and Wilkens.

National Research Council. (2007). *Nutrient Requirements of Horses* (6th ed.). Washington: The National Academies Press.

NOTES:

Laboratory 3
ACTIVITY

Before coming to lab review a minimum of two articles that cover pasture management suggestions. Bring the articles to lab and in a group of 2–3 students make a list of the five most important management aspects. Appoint a group recorder/spokesperson to share and discuss your group's list with the other groups.

Supplemental Activity
PASTURE EVALUATION

Materials:

- Pasture
- Paper & writing utensil

Objective:

The idea is to have students use knowledge they have learned in lab and apply it to a real physical place.

Activity:

1. Come up with a list of ten important characteristics of pastures for horses.
   These ten can be the same as the ones you will list for question 1 of the lab assignment.

2. Find a pasture.

3. Contact the owner of the property to set up an appropriate time to evaluate the pasture.

4. Determine the size of the pasture using an odometer, trundle wheel, or by simply pacing it out.

5. Go out into the pasture to evaluate it based on the ten characteristics you came up with in Number 1.

6. Create a list of positive characteristics of the pasture.

7. Create a second list of items that could be improved about the pasture.

8. ***Thank the landowner for their time and the use of their pasture!***

NOTES:

Name_____

Lab Section_____

Lab Assignment 3
PASTURES FOR HORSES

1. List and briefly describe at least ten items that come to mind when thinking about important characteristics of pastures for horses. Example: location—this affects ease of turnout and ability to observe horses for health and safety reasons.

2. Based on the class discussion and on the information presented in the references for this lab, write a concise summary of important factors involved with pasture management. Include a minimum of five management factors in your summary.

3. Recommend the number of mature horses to put on an area of land in central New York State, measuring 500 ft by 1000 ft in order for the horses to receive adequate nutritional value (during the pasture season). Justify your recommendation. Keep in mind that forage yields within a pasture may decrease as the season progresses from spring through the summer months.

4. Research a pasture seed mix that is marketed to horse owners. Provide the following information:
    Brand
    Weight
    Cost
    Suggested application rate
    Mixture of plant seeds contained
    What type of horse (maintenance, growing, performance, breeding, etc.) is this recommended for and why?

Challenge questions:

1. You have been hired to design a pasture system for a person that has purchased a 150 acre piece of land and intends to build a barn and all needed facilities to support 40 horses. The horses are a combination of boarders and personally-owned lesson horses (by the owner). The goal of the new owner is to have adequate pasture and turnout for all horses while keeping the process of turnout as simple and as efficient as possible. Describe and illustrate how you would design a pasture system. Include items that would be necessary for maintenance. Cite all references used for this question. Please answer this question on a separate page.

2. You own 10 acres of pasture land in the northeast United States and five horses. Research methods of rotational pasture management and then propose a system by which your 10 acres could be utilized most efficiently in a rotational system. Include suggestions for forage species to use and types of fencing to consider. What are other important considerations for this type of pasture system? Since you are in the northeast, you will not have access to 12-month grazing value from your pasture. Please answer this question on a separate page. Diagrams are encouraged. Cite all references.

NOTES:

Laboratory 4
FORAGE 2: HAY FOR HORSES

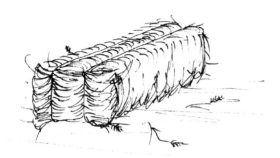

Source: Rachel Monticelli-Turner.

Introduction:

Hay goes with horses. While it varies according to the types of forages used and the form in which it is presented, a common understanding among most U.S. horse owners is that hay is an essential and economical source of nutrients and fiber for horses.

Objectives:

When finished with the material from this laboratory, the student should be able to:

1. Define hay.
2. Describe the process of making forage into hay.
3. Discuss the differences between cuttings of hay (1st, 2nd, etc.).
4. List and describe five criteria in judging the quality of hay.
5. Describe the process of having hay sampled and analyzed.
6. Describe how one would interpret the results of a forage analysis.
7. Demonstrate how to determine the body weight of a horse and suggest an appropriate amount of forage intake based on its body weight.
8. Describe important nutritional concerns related to a variety of forages.

Questions for further discussion:

1. What determines the choice of bale type and size when making hay?
2. Under what circumstances would long-stemmed hay be inappropriate to feed to horses and what are alternatives that could be used?
3. How much money should a horse owner budget for a year's supply of hay?

NOTES:

Manual of Equine Nutrition and Feeding Management, First Edition.
Carol Z. Buckhout and Barbara E. Lindberg.
© 2022 John Wiley & Sons, Inc. Published 2022 by John Wiley & Sons, Inc.
Companion website: www.wiley.com/go/buckhout/manual

NOTES:

Hay

A. Definition: Dried forage (less than 20% moisture) that provides nutrient value to the animals to which it is fed (Lewis, 1996).

B. Types of hay
   1. Legume hays
      a. alfalfa (lucerne)
      b. clover (ladino is the preferred variety)
      c. others: birdsfoot trefoil, lespedeza, etc., this depends on location
   2. Grass hays
      a. timothy
      b. orchard grass
      c. brome grass
      d. rye grass
      e. reed canary grass
      f. bluegrass
      g. others
   3. Cereal grain hays
      a. oat hay
      b. barley hay
      c. others
   4. Mixed hays may be comprised of combinations of legume, grass, and even cereal grain hay

C. Advantages of hay
   1. It is a natural feedstuff and healthy for horses.
   2. It is an economical source of nutrients for the horse.
   3. It can provide significant amounts of nutrients.
   4. It can provide many more nutrients on a dry matter basis than pasture.
   5. Normal cecal and large colon digestive activity depends on forage, such as hay.
   6. It is an economical form of forage to store.

D. Disadvantages of hay
   1. Hay is a difficult product to properly produce (harvest and bale) in order to maximize its nutrient content.
   2. Hay production is labor-intensive.
   3. Nutrient losses in field and in storage may occur.
   4. Improperly cured (dried) hay is a fire hazard due to spontaneous combustion.
   5. Poor-quality hay may contain weeds and other contaminants and may also contain mold, all of which are detrimental to the health of the horse.
   6. A proper storage area is needed in order to maintain the nutrient content.

E. Cuttings of hay

   1. The most nutritious hay comes from forages that are cut at immature stages:

      a. legumes: 1/10th bloom ensures highest level of nutrients

      b. grasses: boot stage (the head is just emerging from the stem) indicates optimum quality.

   2. Nutrient content of cuttings in the Northeastern United States for hay grown for horses:

      a. First cutting: Forages grown for horse hay are generally harvested between early June and mid July as this allows for maximum yield. However, later cutting dates with increased yield may suffer from a declining nutritional content. Variables, especially the weather, affect when first cutting occurs. When forage quality is extremely important to livestock, such as dairy cattle, first cutting is done sooner, beginning as early as mid-May. However, this forage may be used for silage as opposed to baled hay since drying (or curing) early cut forage for hay is very challenging.

      b. Second cutting: The timing of second cutting is directly dependent on when the first cutting was completed and on the growing conditions that occurred between first and second cutting. When a mixed seeding of grasses and legumes is involved, second cutting has a higher quantity of legumes due to the warmer and dryer weather. Yet, while quality of second cutting hay may be greater than first cutting, its yield is usually lower. A five- to six-week period between cuttings is usually recommended, making dates for second cutting for horse hay range from mid-July through late August.

      c. Third cutting: This is a rather unusual occurrence for horse hay in the northeast U.S., but a common occurrence for hay grown in other parts of the country especially for livestock such as dairy and beef animals. Third cutting usually has a nutritional content between that of first and second cutting. Factors that affect the potential of getting a third cutting include moisture, heat, and length of daylight, all of which can be variable in late summer.

      d. Later cuttings: These are strictly dependent on location and weather conditions. In southern and western areas of the U.S., it's possible to get multiple cuttings of hay before the growing conditions require a period of rest for forage plants to re-establish themselves.

An "old school" of thought is that hay for horses does not have to be as nutritious as that for other livestock, such as dairy animals. Therefore, sometimes hay that is of lesser quality is referred to as "horse hay" to denote that it is adequate for horses, but may not have the nutrient content that would be desired for lactating dairy animals. The most important characteristics of any hay for horses is that it be clean and devoid of any dust or mold. Oddly enough, dairy animals can actually withstand small amounts of mold in their forages!

In areas of the western United States where forage is grown by irrigation, forage may be grown and harvested for hay on a continual basis.

NOTES:

e. The number of cuttings is controlled by climate: Forage grown for hay in the northern U.S. requires adequate time for regrowth of the plant before a killing frost. The regrowth ensures that adequate root supply is available to the plant to protect it during the winter, to keep the plant from heaving from the soil when the frost leaves the ground in the spring and to allow growth during the following season to continue.

3. Costs associated with hay cuttings:

a. First cutting: This is usually the least expensive cutting of hay since the nutrient content and quality are assumed to be the lowest.

b. Second and later cuttings: These may be more expensive than first cutting since the nutrient content and quality are generally higher than first cutting.

c. All cuttings: Prices will vary with the location in the country where the hay was produced, how far the hay had to be transported, the size of the bale, and the quality of the forages included in the bale. Hay is usually priced on a per ton basis, but it's not unusual that a horse owner can buy hay that has been priced by the individual bale.

F. Bale size and shape

1. Rectangular bales: These are the traditional forms of baled hay. They generally range in weight from 40 to 80 pounds and the weight is determined by the calibration of the baler. Producing and storing rectangular bales can be very labor-intensive, but equipment is now available that allows the hay producer to be totally hands-off in the baling and storage process.

2. Round bales: This shape and size has become popular with hay producers since they are a more efficient bale to produce. Round bales are large and heavy, with an average diameter of 4–5 feet and an average weight of 900–1200 pounds. They require special equipment for producing and moving them. Horse owners that use round bales must be aware of the potential for moldy forage to exist in the insides of the bales. This can be a real problem given the potential of a horse contracting botulism. Round bales with quality forage are a convenient way to supplement waning pasture forage for a group of horses. Storage of round bales can be challenging due to their size and difficulty in moving them around.

3. Large square or rectangular bales: While these present another option in shape, they have similar properties and precautions to round bales.

G. Judging hay (Gibbs, 2005)
   1. Maturity: A minimal presence of blossoms (in legumes) or relatively small seed heads (in grasses) indicate that the forage was cut at an immature stage. Also the dark joints present in the stems of grasses lighten as the plants age.

   2. Texture: Soft and pliable stems indicate less mature plants than coarse and tough stems.

   3. Foreign matter: A lack of weeds, debris, mold, and dust.

   4. Leafiness: The higher the percentage of leaves, the higher the nutrient content.

   5. Color: Bright green is the best indicator of forage quality; bleached or brown indicate nutrient losses during storage or the use of overly mature plants at the time of making hay.

Steps in judging hay
   1. Observe visually for the above criteria.
   2. Smell the hay for mold and dust.
   3. Feel the texture.
   4. Lift a bale: A heavy bale may contain mold or other foreign matter. Lightness may indicate older bales and a lack of nutrients.
   5. Cut open a bale. The flakes should pull apart readily and should smell sweet and fresh.

H. Determining the nutrient content of hay and other forages
   Visual inspection of hay can give one a general idea of its quality. Items such as rich color or abundant leaves indicate good quality while a faded color and a high percentage of stems means it's of poorer quality. Knowing the specific nutrient content of forage is very useful to enhance a horse's health and to optimize its performance. This process goes beyond a visual inspection as it involves obtaining a representative sample of the forage and having it chemically analyzed in a laboratory. Referred to as a forage analysis, horse owners, and managers are more routinely using this procedure to fine tune their equine diets.

   1. The sampling process: Providing a representative sample is the most important part of the sampling process (Equi-Analytical Laboratories procedures for taking a hay sample, n.d.).

       a. The most thorough way to sample hay is to obtain core samples by using a hay corer, also called a hay probe. This device resembles a large drill that is designed to bore lengthwise through the center of a bale of hay and cut the plant matter in uniform pieces, approximately 1″ in length. The resulting product is called a core sample.

NOTES:

Equine metabolic syndrome:

Plant researchers have developed some cool season grass forages with improved energy content. This has been especially beneficial for production animals such as dairy cattle. However, the energy found mostly in the form of fructans or "forage sugars" can negatively impact horses. Fructans are degraded in the cecum where the end products can upset the harmony of the fiber fermenting microbes. Health implications from forages containing high fructan levels include laminitis and obesity. Horses with specific metabolic issues such as insulin resistance, Pituitary Pars Intermedia Dysfunction (Equine Cushing's disorder) or poly-saccharide storage myopathy will have very specific dietary requirements and the fructan levels of their diets must be very low. Cool season grass forages include: timothy, orchard grass, Kentucky bluegrass, and brome grass. Management of the diets of horses prone to equine metabolic syndrome can be a challenge.

    b.   By sampling approximately 20 bales of hay, combining the samples together and then packaging a partial amount of the mixture for the analysis, the best possible analysis may be obtained.

    c.   Laboratories that are designed to analyze feeds generally provide a sampling package, instructions, and often the sample may be sent through the mail to the laboratory.

    d.   Results may be returned through the mail, faxed, or provided through e-mail. It is not unusual that analysis results may be obtained within 24 hours after the sample has left the farm.

    e.   Horse owners may also want to have an idea of the nutrient content of their pastures. For an accurate result a representative sample is needed. Using scissors, the horse owner may cut samples of forage from at least 20 different areas of the pasture at the level that the horse would be grazing. Before mailing, the sample should be frozen overnight to halt the respiration of the plants.

2.   Interpreting results of a forage analysis: Knowing the specific nutrient content of a forage will allow some fine-tuning of an equine diet. A forage with a higher than expected crude protein content may mean that less protein will need to be provided in the form of grain. A higher than average NDF would indicate that digestible energy needs to be provided from another source, such as grain or beet pulp. The sugar content of forages, evaluated as water soluble carbohydrates (WSC) and ethanol soluble carbohydrates (ESC), is an important measure since horses are increasingly susceptible to forms of equine metabolic syndrome such as insulin resistance. Also, the level of minerals and vitamins is useful in determining whether a horse should be receiving a supplemental source of specific minerals or vitamins.

3.   Challenges with forage analyses: Horse owners may not have the tools or the knowledge to have their forages sampled and analyzed. Some feed companies provide analyses as a courtesy for their clients. Cooperative Extension professionals might provide the equipment and the personnel to assist with both the sampling process and with interpreting the results. The forage analysis laboratories may provide sampling and interpretation tips. There are numerous articles available about the importance and process of forage analysis. The Equi-Analytical laboratory, based in Ithaca, NY, is one of the largest feed analysis labs in the country. Their website, www.equi-analytical.com, is full of useful information about obtaining and interpreting a forage analysis, including a glossary of nutrient terms.

Formulas to estimate body weight in pounds:

Since a horse's daily feed intake is based on a percentage of its body weight then one needs to have some idea of what their horse actually does weigh. This can be accomplished through a variety of methods. Certainly, the best and most accurate method would be to have a livestock scale in the barn. However, since these tend to be rather expensive, most horse owners opt for a different method. A weight tape, which looks much like a measuring tape, converts the distance around the horse's heart girth into pounds (or kilograms). Also, several formulas are available that convert a combination of heart girth and body length measurements into weight. Examples of these formulas are listed below. No matter what method is used, the consistency of how it is used is the most important part.

a. mature horses:

$$\frac{(\text{heart girth, in inches})^2 \times (\text{body length in inches})}{330} = \text{Body weight in pounds}$$

b. yearlings:

$$\frac{(\text{heart girth, in inches})^2 \times (\text{body length in inches})}{301} = \text{Body weight in pounds}$$

c. weanlings:

$$\frac{(\text{heart girth, in inches})^2 \times (\text{body length in inches})}{280} = \text{Body weight in pounds}$$

d. miniature horses:

$$(9.36 \times \text{heart girth in inches}) + (5.01 \times \text{length in inches}) - 348.53 = \text{Body weight in pounds}$$

Sources:

a. adapted from: Gibbs, n.d.

b. adapted from: Hathaway, 2007.

c. adapted from Hathaway, 2007.

d. adapted from Kentucky Equine Research, 2002.

For additional information:

West, C., (2008, May). Fiber in hay: What's the magic number? *The Horse*. Retrieved from https://thehorse.com/122330/ fiber-in-hay-whats-the-magic-number/.

References:

Equi-Analytical Laboratories. (n.d.). *Procedures for taking a hay sample*. Retrieved from https://equi-analytical.com/ feed-and-forage-analysis/taking-a-sample/.

Gibbs, P. (2005). *Selection and use of hay and processed roughage in horse feeding*. Retrieved from Texas A&M University AgriLIFE Extension: https://animalscience.tamu.edu/wp-content/uploads/sites/14/2012/04/nutrition-selection-and-use-of-roughage-in-horses.pdf.

Hathaway, M. (2007). *Feeding the Weanling and Yearling Horse*. Retrieved from the University of Minnesota Extension website: https://extension.umn.edu/horse-nutrition/feeding-weanling-and-yearling-horse.

Kentucky Equine Research staff. (2002). Feeding the Miniature Horse. Retrieved from Equinews: https://ker.com/equinews/ feeding-miniature-horse/.

Lewis, L. (1996). *Feeding and Care of the Horse* (2nd ed.). Me dia, PA: Lippincott, Williams and Wilkens.

Laboratory 4
ACTIVITIES

1. Participate in the process of sampling hay for a forage analysis. Review a forage analysis report and define the categories of nutrients that are found on the report.

2. Examine several bales of hay and rate each of them for the characteristics listed below on a scale of 1–3, where 1 = poor; 2 = good and 3 = excellent. Total your ratings and compare them with other classmates. Speculate how the ratings would compare to the information on a forage analysis.

Maturity: _____   _____   _____

Texture: _____   _____   _____

Foreign matter: _____   _____   _____

Leafiness: _____   _____   _____

Color: _____   _____   _____

3. Guess the weight of your assigned horse. Apply the appropriate weight formula and utilize a weight tape. If a livestock scale is available, compare the horse's weight with what you found from the formula and the weight tape.

Guess: _____

Weight tape: _____

Formula: _____

Scale: _____

Supplemental Activity
SCAVENGER HUNT

Materials:

- Tape
- Paper & writing utensil

Objective:

The purpose of this activity is to further familiarize the student with which portion of the plant is the seed head and the differences between plant species.

Activity:

1. Visit your assigned horse and look at their hay.

2. Determine the types of plants found within the hay.

3. Tape a seed head from every type of grass found onto your paper.

4. Label each seed head with the type of grass.

Name_____

Lab Section_____

Lab 4 Assignment
HAY FOR HORSES

1. Discuss the pros and cons of feeding first and second cutting to horses. Include economic factors in your answer.

2. The actual amount of hay to feed per day is a common question. Research this topic and summarize your findings. Remember that horse intakes are based as a percent of their body weight. Cite all sources used to answer this question.

3. Review the appearances and important characteristics of each of the forages listed on the following pages and, when appropriate, include a health concern that they might pose. State whether each is a legume or a grass (when not obvious) in the Appearance and Characteristics section. (Useful reference: Lewis, 1996, pp.108–110.)

Forage	Appearance & Characteristics	Possible Health Concern
a. alfalfa		
b. birdsfoot trefoil		
c. alsike clover		
d. crimson clover		
e. red clover		
f. sweet clover		
g. white clover		
h. ladino clover		
i. lespedeza		
j. crown vetch		
k. tall fescue		

Forage	Appearance & Characteristics	Possible Health Concern
l. orchard grass		
m. brome grass		
n. bermuda grass		
o. digit grasses and bahia grass		
p. bluegrass		
q. reed canary grass		
r. timothy		
s. rye grass		
t. sorghum and sudan grass		
u. millet		

NOTES:

Laboratory 5
CONCENTRATES FOR HORSES

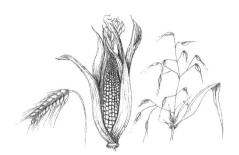

Source: Rachel Monticelli-Turner.

Introduction:

The purpose of this laboratory is to provide information about the properties and characteristics of concentrates. These high energy feeds are commonly referred to as grains. Since forages cannot always provide adequate levels of nutrients needed by high performing horses, grains are supplied to boost the nutritional level of a horse's diet. Often grains are grown and processed for human consumption. The "leftovers" that occur from the processing methods also make very useful horse feed ingredients. These are called by-product feeds and will be further explored in Laboratory 6.

Objectives:

When finished with the material from this laboratory, the student should be able to:

1. Identify samples of natural concentrates and state what nutrient they all share in common.
2. Define the term "by-product" feed.
3. Explain why some concentrates are mechanically processed for use in horse feeds and list six methods of processing feeds.
4. Describe the three required items of information found on commercial feed labels.
5. Discuss guidelines for feeding concentrates to horses.
6. Describe the Henneke Body Condition Scoring System and tell why it's useful for determining concentrate needs of horses.

Questions for further discussion:

1. What factors cause the variations in prices of concentrates in different regions of the country?
2. What concentrates tend to be the most popular to use in horse diets?

General overview

While many horses require grain to balance their nutritional needs, it should be also noted that some horses may not need grain in their diets. Horses that are under high physical demands or are in an important life phase such as growth or lactation need the additional nutrients that are provided by concentrates. However, horses that are fully grown and are not under great physical demands may perform very well without added grain in their diets. The goal of this laboratory is to familiarize the student with the nature and variety of concentrates and to understand when concentrates should be provided in the equine diet.

Manual of Equine Nutrition and Feeding Management, First Edition.
Carol Z. Buckhout and Barbara E. Lindberg.
© 2022 John Wiley & Sons, Inc. Published 2022 by John Wiley & Sons, Inc.
Companion website: www.wiley.com/go/buckhout/manual

NOTES:

NOTES:

A. Definition

Concentrates include the seed portion of plants or the by-products derived from the seeds. Their nutrient content is more consistent and more compact than forages and they are considered to be a concentrated source of nutrients. The term "grain" is used interchangeably with the term "concentrate."

B. Characteristics

1. All concentrates are high in energy content (1.1 Mcal/lb or 2.42 Mcal/kg of DE and higher) (NRC, 2007).
2. Concentrates are low in fiber content (less than 18% crude fiber).
3. Concentrates *may* be a source of protein, some minerals, and some vitamins.
4. Concentrates are generally more expensive than forages.

C. Classification

1. Low protein (cereal grains): less than 20% crude protein examples: oats, corn, barley, sorghum, wheat, rye, rice, millet, emmer, spelt, and triticale.
2. Moderate protein (20–30% crude protein) and high protein (greater than 30% crude protein): these are essentially by-product feeds in which the nutrient content, especially the protein content, has been altered. Examples include corn distillers' grains, corn gluten feed, soybean meal, linseed meal, and others. This area will be further explored in Laboratory 6.

D. Processed concentrate feeds

1. Processing changes the physical form of the feed to make the feed more digestible.
2. Examples (review definitions of any unfamiliar terms)
   a. crimping
   b. grinding
   c. cracking
   d. de-hulling
   e. rolling
   f. roasting
   g. drying
   h. pelleting
   i. extruding

E. Feeding grain to horses: suggestions and rules of thumb

1. Since grains have a more concentrated amount of nutrients when compared to forages, the amount of grain in the diets of horses should be monitored closely.
2. A general thumb rule: The amount of grain fed to a horse should not exceed half of the total daily intake by weight. Exceptions include: nursing foals, weanlings, and horses under a high degree of exercise, such as race horses.

3. Most concentrates fed to horses come in a blended group of feeds referred to as a grain mix. Grain mixes are formulated by nutritional experts and different formulations may provide for needs of different classes of horses (maintenance, growing, breeding, or various levels of activity).

4. The form of the concentrate may vary depending on the combination of feeds included and the type of animal being fed (ex: young or aged); forms include sweet feeds (with molasses to blend feeds together), pelleted feeds (one cannot distinguish the individual feed ingredients), and extruded feeds (less-dense than pelleted feeds after going through the extrusion process).

5. Complete feeds are high-fiber mixes which combine typical grains (natural or by-products) and source(s) of fiber, such as alfalfa meal, beet pulp, and soy hulls. Complete feeds may be processed in pelleted or extruded forms.

6. Limit the amount of grain fed in a single feeding to a maximum of 5 pounds (Lewis, 1996).

7. Always read the feed label on all purchased grains for feeding instructions and other important information.

8. One can have grains analyzed for their nutritional value. This would be especially useful when feeding single grains (such as oats) that have been purchased from a local source.

References:

Hennecke, D.R., Potter, G.D., Kreider, J.L., Yeates, B.F. (1983). Relationship between condition score, physical measurements and the body fat percentage in mares. *Equine Veterinary Journal*, 15 (4), 371–372.

Lewis, L. (1996). *Feeding and Care of the Horse* (2nd ed.). Media, PA: Lippincott, Williams and Wilkens.

National Research Council. (2007). *Nutrient Requirements of Horses* (6th ed.). Washington: The National Academies Press.

Henneke Body Condition Scoring System

Body condition scoring is important to determine how overweight or underweight an individual horse may be.

To properly assign a condition score to a horse the neck, withers, loin, tail head, ribs, and shoulder of a horse need to be evaluated.

Body condition scores range from 1 to 9 and are as follows:

1
Poor

2
Very Thin

3
Thin

4
Moderately Thin

5
Moderate

6
Moderately Fleshy

7
Fleshy

8
Fat

9
Extremely Fat

Source: Henneke, et. al. 1983

NOTES:

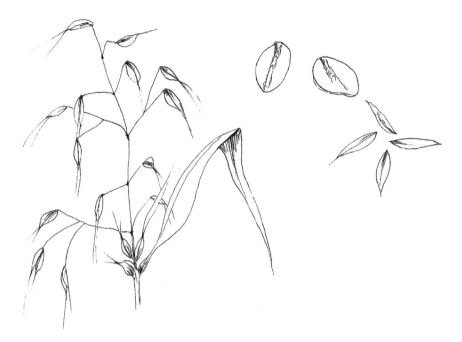

Figure 5.1 Oats: *Avena sativa.* *Source: Rachel Monticelli-Turner.*

*Please note that figures are
not drawn to the same scale.*

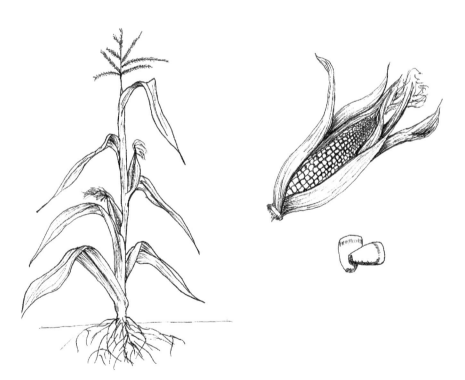

Figure 5.2 Corn: *Zea mays.* *Source: Rachel Monticelli-Turner.*

NOTES:

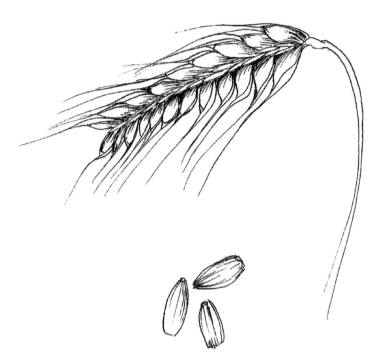

Figure 5.3 Barley: *Hordeum vulgare.* *Source: Rachel Monticelli-Turner.*

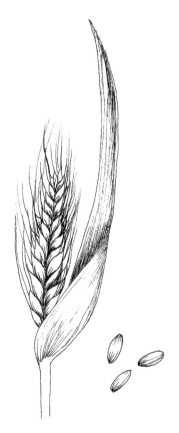

Figure 5.4 Wheat: *Triticum aestivum.*
Source: Rachel Monticelli-Turner.

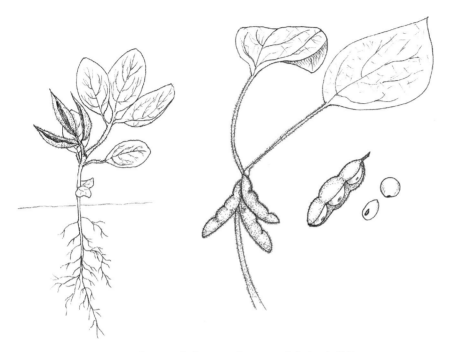

Figure 5.5 Soybeans: *Glycine max.* Source: *Rachel Monticelli-Turner.*

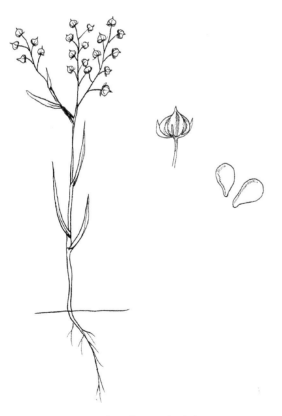

Figure 5.6 Flax: *Linum usitatissimum.*
Source: *Rachel Monticelli-Turner.*

NOTES:

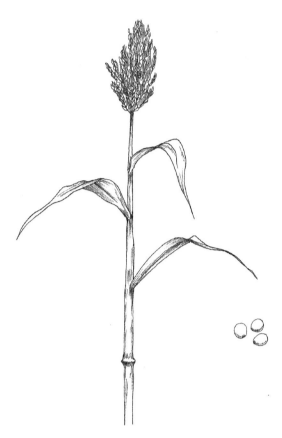

Figure 5.7* Sorghum: *Sorghum bicolor.
Source: *Rachel Monticelli-Turner.*

Laboratory 5
ACTIVITIES

1. Feed labels: Complete the exercises below. Use the examples of feed labels provided on the next pages for assistance.

    a. List and describe the major categories of information that must be provided on a feed label by the feed manufacturer.

    b. What are some typical types of concentrates that might be found in a grain mix? List examples and indicate whether they are natural feeds or by-product feeds and whether they have been processed.

2. Observe the concentrate illustrations and samples, if provided, for both their plant and seed forms. Make note of their identifying shape, color, and texture. Record your observations.

Manetain

This feed was designed to be used to maintain adult horses.

Guaranteed Analysis:

Crude Protein	Min	10.0	%		
Crude Fat	Min	4.0	%		
Crude Fiber	Max	10.00	%		
Calcium	Min	0.65	%	Max	1.05 %
Phosphorus	Min	0.50	%		
Copper	Min	34.00	PPM		
Manganese	Min	108.50	PPM		
Selenium	Min	0.40	PPM		
Zinc	Min	120.00	PPM		
Vitamin A	Min	5,000.00	IU/lb		

Ingredients:

Steam Flaked Corn, Coarse Cracked Corn, Steam Crimped Oats, Cane Molasses, Wheat Middlings, Soybean Hulls, Ground Corn, Vegetable Oil, Salt, Calcium Carbonate, Calcium Sulfate, Monocalcium Phosphate, Zinc Sulfate, Copper Sulfate, Manganese Sulfate, Copper Proteinate, Manganese Proteinate, Calcium Propionate, Cobalt Carbonate, Calcium Iodate, Ferrous Sulfate, Sodium Selenite, Selenium Yeast, Vitamin E Supplement, Vitamin A Supplement, Vitamin D3 Supplement, Choline Chloride, Riboflavin, Niacin, Folic Acid, Biotin, Vitamin B12 Supplement, Thiamine Mononitrate, Pyridoxine Hydrochloride, Menadione Sodium Bisulfite Complex (Source of Vitamin K Activity), Oat Mill By-product, L-Ascorbyl-2-Polyphosphate (Source of Vitamin C), DL-Methionine

***Warning: Do not feed to sheep because it contains supplemental copper.

Product Code: 8675309_JT2
Net Wt. 50 LB
Manufactured by:
College Feeds: A Smart Decision
Main Office
Cazenovia, NY, 13035

Lot: 006

Figure 5.8 Example of a feed label . Source: Sara Tanner Mastellar, Ph.D.

Scholar Horse Feed

This feed was designed to be fed to the average school horse.

Guaranteed Analysis:

Crude Protein	Min	13.00	%			
Crude Fat	Min	6.00	%			
Crude Fiber	Max	8.00	%			
Calcium	Min	1.00	%	Max	1.20	%
Phosphorus	Min	0.85	%			
Copper	Min	51.00	PPM			
Selenium	Min	0.70	PPM			
Zinc	Min	159.00	PPM			
Vitamin A	Min	3985.30	IU/LB			

Ingredients:

Processed Grain By-Products, Grain Products, Roughage Products, Forage Products, Soybean Meal, Calcium Carbonate, Molasses Products, Plant Protein Products, Salt, Lysine, Methionine Supplement, Natural and Artificial Preservatives, Potassium Chloride, Sodium Selenite, Primaiac, L-Threonine, Zinc Sulfate, Natural & Artificial Flavors added, Copper Sulfate, Selenium Yeast, Selenium, Folic Acid, Zinc Amino Acid Complex, Manganese Supplement, Riboflavin Supplement, Biotin, Thiamine Supplement, Vitamin E Supplement, Vitamin D3 Supplement, Vitamin B12 Supplement, Magnesium Oxide, Cobalt Carbonate, Ferrous Sulfate, Manganese Sulfate, Copper Chloride, Zinc Oxide

***Warning: Do not fed to sheep because it contains supplemental copper.

Product Code: 15638752_THY
Net Wt. 50 LB

Manufactured by:
Scholar Horse Feeds: A Smart Decision
Main Office
Cazenovia, NY, 13035

Lot: 008

Figure 5.9 Example of a feed label. Source: Sara Tanner Mastellar, Ph.D.

Supplemental Activity
AN EXERCISE IN DESCRIPTION

Materials:

- Index cards or slips of paper
- Partners
- Blindfold (optional)
- Stopwatch (optional)

Objective:

The objective of this activity is to increase the students' ability to describe feeds to other, less knowledgeable, individuals. This activity will also increase familiarity with different samples provided in lab.

Activity:

Pretend you are across the country looking at a hunter prospect. Your flight back has been delayed. Luckily you get a hold of your neighbor and they agree to feed your horses. Unfortunately, your grain bins are not labeled.

1. Write descriptions of the samples provided in lab as if you were describing them over the phone to your neighbor on index cards or slips of paper. Write the name of the feed on the back.

2. Shuffle the cards or slips of paper.

3. Hand the cards to your partner and see how many feeds he/she can identify based on your descriptions.

4. Switch roles and try your hand at identifying the feeds based on your partner's descriptions of them.

5. For a harder version of this activity blindfold your partner and describe the feed to them verbally. Use a stopwatch to see how fast you can get your partner to guess correctly. Compete with other pairs for the fastest time.

Name_____

Lab Section_____

Lab 5 Assignment
CONCENTRATES FOR HORSES

1. What basic nutritional property is common to ALL concentrates? _____

2. Complete the following chart. Useful reference: NRC, 2007, Table 16-6. Use this chart as a study guide for a potential feeds identification quiz.

Feed	DE (Mcal/kg)	CP %	Reasons for Feeding	Possible Precautions
a. Barley, grain, rolled				
b. Corn grain, cracked, dry				
c. Corn grain, ground, dry				
d. Corn, grain, steam-flaked				
e. Oats, grain, rolled				
f. Oats, grain, whole, 32/lb per bu				
g. Oats, grain, whole, 38/lb per bu				
h. Soybean Seeds, whole				
i. Soybean, Seeds, whole heated				
j. Wheat Grain, rolled				

3. Discuss the outdated term "total digestible nutrients" (TDN) as opposed to the newer, more accurate term "digestible energy" (DE) with regard to how they both measure the energy value of a feed. Include the units in which they measure energy.

Challenge question:

1. Suggest two different situations when one would need to feed grain to horses and suggest how to determine the amount and the frequency of feeding the grain (cite references).

Laboratory 6
(1) BY-PRODUCT FEEDS AND ADDITIVES
(2) THE CONCEPTS OF "AS SAMPLED" AND "DRY MATTER"

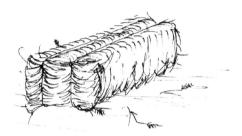

Source: Rachel Monticelli-Turner.

Introduction:

This exercise has two purposes:

1. To further explore the use of non-forage products in the horse's diet in the form of by-product feeds and feed additives. Both are intended to enhance the nutritional value of the ration.

2. To enable the student to learn how to compare feeds on two different basis: (1) the *as sampled* basis, which accounts for any water contained in the feed and (2) the *dry matter* basis, a theoretical concept of removing the water content from feeds. Understanding these concepts enables a true comparison of different feeds that have different moisture contents, such as pasture versus hay. Some feed composition tables provide the nutrient content on an *as sampled* basis, yet other tables provide the nutrient composition on a *dry matter* basis. A student of nutrition should know the difference between *as sampled* and *dry matter*.

Objectives:

When finished with the material from this laboratory, the student should be able to:

1. Define and give examples of by-product feeds made from grains.
2. Define and give examples of feed additives.
3. Explain the difference between as sampled and dry matter.
4. Calculate the amount of dry matter in a feed.
5. Convert a quantity of dry matter to an as sampled basis.

Questions for further discussion:

1. What are some of the most popular by-product feeds used in horse grain mixes and why are they used?

2. What are two common additives that can be found in horse grain mixes and why?

Manual of Equine Nutrition and Feeding Management, First Edition.
Carol Z. Buckhout and Barbara E. Lindberg.
© 2022 John Wiley & Sons, Inc. Published 2022 by John Wiley & Sons, Inc.
Companion website: www.wiley.com/go/buckhout/manual

By-product feeds

A major reason that grains are grown in the world is to process products for human consumption and use. Examples include flour, cereals, and fuel. There may be left-over portions of grain from processing and these can make excellent animal feeds. These left-over feeds are called by-product feeds.

Suggested categories of by-product feeds may include:

1. Plant by-products

    a. Low protein (less than 20% crude protein)—good sources of digestible fiber (NRC, 2007)

        examples: wheat bran, oat hulls, beet pulp

    b. Moderate protein (20–30% crude protein) (NRC, 2007)

        examples: distillers' grains, corn gluten feed

    c. High protein (more than 30% crude protein) (NRC, 2007)

        examples: soybean meal, linseed meal, corn gluten meal (some may be deficient in essential amino acids)

2. Fats and oils

    a. Plant sources: rice bran, corn oil

    b. Animal sources: tallow (however, animal fats and oils are much less stable and more prone to rancidity than plant oils)

3. Animal by-products—excellent high-quality protein sources, but are generally not used in commercial concentrates because:

    a. They can reduce the shelf life of the feeds in which they are found.

    b. There have been concerns regarding disease resulting from ingestion of infected animal by-products.
        Examples: bone meal, meat meal, fish meal.

Feed additives

A feed additive is a product that enhances the nutritional value of a diet by increasing some aspect of the diet from palatability to digestive properties. These products tend to be manufactured as opposed to being natural products. They must be proven safe in order to be marketed in the United States (Lewis, 1996).

The assignment for this lab exercise will provide the opportunity to explore and study the nutritional properties of common by-product feeds used in horse rations as well as various feed additives.

As sampled and dry matter conversions

General overview:

Every feed contains a certain amount of water; the non-water portion of the feed is termed the **dry matter**. A high-moisture feed, such as pasture or silage, contains a larger amount of water and less **dry matter** per pound as compared to a drier feed, such as hay (which contains a small amount of water and more dry matter per pound). The term **as sampled** (or "as fed") refers to the whole feed (**dry matter** and water) (Equi-analytical Laboratories, n.d.).

Except for water, the nutrients in a feed are found in the **dry matter** portion. Therefore, when one is working with feeds of varying moisture contents, the **dry matter** becomes a basis for comparison. Review the graphs below that represent different feeds. As the moisture contents vary, it would be very difficult to compare the amounts of nutrients contained in the feeds without converting all feeds to a **dry matter** basis.

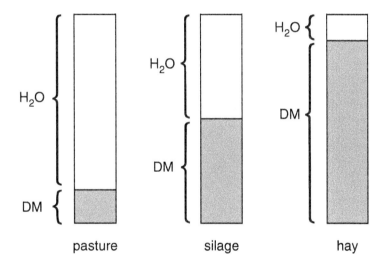

Figure 6.1 As sampled feed.
Source: Laurie Gilmore Selleck.

The terms "as fed" and "as sampled" can be used interchangeably. This is done throughout the remainder of this lab manual.

When multiplying or dividing with percentages, remember to convert the percentage to its decimal form.

Examples:
89% = 0.89
0.35% = 0.0035
2.5% = 0.025

Examples of calculations between as sampled and dry matter

Generic algebraic equation:

$$\frac{\%}{100} = \frac{part}{whole}$$

In order to use the algebraic equation above for example 1, determine the number for each variable. In this case:

% = 90

part = x (this is what we want to find)

whole = 20

$$\frac{90}{100} = \frac{x}{20}$$

Solving for x will give us our answer of 18 lb.

1. Convert an as sampled amount of feed to its dry matter amount:

General rule:

The amount of feed (as sampled) × the % dry matter of the feed = the amount of dry matter in the feed

Example:

A forage analysis indicates that a sample of first cutting hay contained 90% dry matter and 10% water. How many pounds of dry matter would be found in 20 pounds of this hay?

Answer:

20 lb × 0.90 = 18 lb dry matter

To find the answer apply the general rule or the algebraic equation.

2. Convert dry matter to as sampled basis:

General rule:

The amount of dry matter ÷ % dry matter of the feed = amount as sampled

Example:

You want to make sure that your horse receives 18 pounds of dry matter to insure that it will receive correct amounts of nutrients. Compare the amount of second cutting hay (88% dry matter) to pasture grass (35% dry matter) that the horse would have to eat in order to receive the 18 pounds of dry matter.

Answer:

$$\text{Second cutting hay}: \frac{18\,\text{lb dry matter}}{0.88} = 20.45\,\text{lb as sampled basis}$$

$$\text{Pasture grass}: \frac{18\,\text{lb dry matter}}{0.35} = 51.4\,\text{lb as sampled basis}$$

Example 2:

Solving the algebraic equation for second cutting:

% = 88

part = 18

whole = x

$$\frac{88}{100} = \frac{18}{x}$$

And for pasture grass:

$$\frac{35}{100} = \frac{18}{x}$$

3. *Dry matter conversions using the metric system:*

Example:

A bale of hay that weighs 23 kilograms was analyzed to contain 88% dry matter content. How many pounds of dry matter are in the bale of hay?

Answer:

Use the rule for converting as sampled to dry matter. When finished, determine how many pounds the bale of hay weighs and how many pounds of dry matter it contains.

23 kg × 0.88 = 20.24 kg dry matter, but the question asks for the answer in pounds, so convert the answer to pounds:

20.24 kg × 2.2 lb / kg = 44.53 lb

Or determine how many pounds the bale of hay weighs first:

23 kg × 2.2 lb / kg = 50.6 lb

And then find the amount of dry matter:

50.6 lb × 0.88 = 44.53 lb

References:

Equi-Analytical Laboratories. (n.d.). *As sampled versus dry matter results.* Retrieved from Equi-Analytical website: https://equi-analytical.com/resources/as-sampled-vs-dry-matter-results/.

Lewis, L. (1996). *Feeding and Care of the Horse* (2nd ed.). Media, PA: Lippincott, Williams and Wilkens.

National Research Council. (2007). *Nutrient Requirements of Horses* (6th ed.). Washington: The National Academies Press.

Converting kilograms (kg) to pounds (lb):

1 kg = 2.2 lb (approximately)

Forage analyses usually report nutrient compositions on both an as sampled (or as fed) and a dry matter basis. The nutrient composition of commercial feeds is generally reported only on an as sampled basis. The dry matter content of commercial feeds is also not reported and can be assumed to be 90%, unless more specific information is given.

Supplemental Activity
TASTY DRY MATTER

Materials:

- Ingredients, utensils, etc. to make cookies
- Balance or postage scale

Objective:

The purpose of this exercise is to solidify the concept of dry matter.

Activity:

1. Make dough for cookies.

2. Weigh a cookie before putting it in the oven.

3. Bake the cookie to remove excess water.

4. Weigh the cookie after it has cooled from baking.

5. Enjoy!

Name_____

Lab Section_____

Laboratory 6 Activity
AS SAMPLED AND DRY MATTER CONVERSIONS

1. Convert the following:

    a.   40 lb hay, as sampled (88% dry matter) =   _____ lb dry matter

    b.   30 lb pasture, as sampled (25% dry matter) =   _____ lb dry matter

    c.   15 lb hay, as sampled (91% dry matter) =   _____ lb dry matter

    d.   12 lb silage, as sampled (52% dry matter) =   _____ lb dry matter

    e.   12 lb hay, dry matter basis, (90% dry matter) =   _____ lb as sampled

    f.   14 lb pasture, dry matter basis (20% dry matter) =   _____ lb as sampled

    g.   10 kilograms hay, as sampled (87% dry matter) =   _____ kg dry matter

                                                                              _____ lb dry matter

    h.   12 kg pasture, dry matter (25% dry matter) =   _____ kg as sampled

                                                                              _____ lb as sample

2. A forage analysis of a sample of timothy hay indicated that it contained 85% dry matter. If 20 pounds are being fed to a horse, how many pounds of dry matter is the horse being fed?

3. A horse is fed the following ration: 12 lb 1st cutting hay (88% dry matter) and 4 lb grain (85% dry matter). How many total pounds of dry matter does the horse receive?

4. Observe samples of by-product feeds provided by your instructor. Make note of the color, texture, and smell of each sample. Keep a list of your observations and use the list when completing question 1 in the assignment section.

NOTES:

Name_____

Lab Section_____

Lab 6 Assignment

(1) BY-PRODUCT FEEDS AND FEED ADDITIVES

(2) AS SAMPLED AND DRY MATTER CONVERSIONS

1. **By-product feeds:** Complete the following chart and use it as a study guide for a potential quiz. Useful references: NRC (2007): Chapter 8 and Table 16-6; Lewis (1996): Chapter 4 and Table 6.

By-product	*Origin/Description*	DE (Mcal/kg)	CP %	*Possible Precautions*
a. Alfalfa meal				
b. Almond hulls				
c. Beet, sugar pulp (unmolassed)				
d. Brewer's grains, dried				
e. Canola meal				
f. Citrus pulp (pomace)				
g. Corn gluten feed				

By-product	Origin/Description	DE (Mcal/kg)	CP %	Possible Precautions
h. Corn gluten meal				
i. Cottonseed meal				
j. Distillers' grains				
k. Linseed meal				
l. Molasses, sugar beet				
m. Oat hulls				
n. Peanut hulls				
o. Peanut seed meal				
p. Rice bran				

By-product	Origin/Description	DE (Mcal/kg)	CP %	Possible Precautions
q. Rice hulls				
r. Soybean hulls				
s. Soybean meal, solv. 44% CP				
t. Sunflower hulls				
u. Sunflower seed meal				
v. Wheat bran				
w. Wheat middlings				

Sources: Based on Lewis (1996), National Research Council (2007).

2. **Feed additives:** Complete the following chart. Useful references: NRC (2007): Chapter 9; Lewis (1996): Chapter 4.

Feed Additive	Origin/Description	Purpose
a. Zeolite		
b. Flavoring agents		
c. Digestion enhancers		
d. Probiotics		
e. Antibiotic feed additives		
f. Mold inhibitors		
g. Antioxidants		

Sources: Based on Lewis (1996), National Research Council (2007).

Dry matter/as sampled questions:
Show your calculations and label all units on your answers.

3. A sample of first cutting hay was analyzed at a forage testing lab. The analysis indicated that the dry matter content of the hay was 91%. You have weighed out 30 pounds of this hay.

   a. How many pounds of dry matter are in the 30 pounds?

   b. How many pounds of water are in the 30 pounds?

4. A sample of second cutting mixed legume hay was analyzed to contain 88% dry matter. One bale of this hay weighs 65 pounds.

   a. How many pounds of dry matter are contained in one bale?

   b. How many pounds of water are contained in one bale?

5. The forage analysis of your pasture indicates that the moisture content is 75% (therefore dry matter is 25%). If your horse eats 20 pounds of the pasture grass in one day, how many pounds of dry matter would the horse consume?

6. You have determined that your horse needs to consume 13 pounds of dry matter from hay in order to receive adequate nutrients per day. Your hay was analyzed to contain 90% dry matter. How many pounds of hay would be required on an as sampled basis?

7. You are doing a comparative study of forages with different moisture contents. If you plan to feed 18 pounds of each forage on a dry matter basis, show how the as sampled amounts vary as moisture content varies:

    a. First cutting mostly grass hay, 86% dry matter

    b. Second cutting mostly legume hay, 90% dry matter

    c. Third cutting mixed grass and legume hay, immature, 84% dry matter

    d. Grass pasture, 22% dry matter

8. You need to feed the following amounts of dry matter (in kilograms) to your horse. Convert these amounts to as sampled and then convert the kg of as sampled to pounds of as sampled.

    a. 10 kg mixed grass hay (89% dry matter)

    b. 2.5 kg sweet feed (90% dry matter)

Laboratory 7
DETERMINING THE NUTRIENT CONTENT OF FEEDS

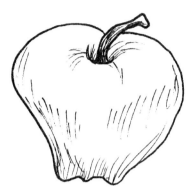

Source: Rachel Monticelli-Turner.

Introduction:

Does the feed that a horse receives provide adequate nutrients to meet its daily nutrient requirements? Knowing how to calculate specific amounts of individual nutrients contained in a feed is a key step to analyzing a diet for a horse. The purpose of this laboratory exercise is to inform students how to determine the quantity of individual nutrients found within a feed.

Objectives:

When finished with the material from this lab the student should be able to:

1. Calculate the amounts of digestible energy, crude protein, calcium, and phosphorus contained in a given amount of feed.
2. Explain why the calculations may be done using the percentages of nutrients on an as sampled basis or on a dry matter basis.

Question for further discussion:

1. What are three factors that can reduce the nutrient content of a feed?

General overview

Feed information from a forage analysis or from a feed label or from a table includes the nutrient content as percentages. Knowing the specific weights of feeds along with the nutrient percentages allows one to calculate the specific amount of nutrients provided by any feed. This information may be used to determine whether a horse's nutritional needs are satisfied.

Manual of Equine Nutrition and Feeding Management, First Edition.
Carol Z. Buckhout and Barbara E. Lindberg.
© 2022 John Wiley & Sons, Inc. Published 2022 by John Wiley & Sons, Inc.
Companion website: www.wiley.com/go/buckhout/manual

NOTES:

NOTES:

Digestible energy (DE) is not specifically included on labels for commercial feeds. However, as the table below shows, the amount of DE is related to the amounts of crude fiber and crude fat within a concentrate mix. Study the chart and note how digestible energy changes in relation to increasing amounts of crude fiber and crude fat.

Table 7.1
Correlations Between Crude Fiber, Crude Fat, and Digestible Energy

Crude Fiber	DE, Mcal/lb (≤5% Crude Fat)	DE, Mcal/lb (>5% Crude Fat)
2%	1.65	1.75
4%	1.55	1.65
6%	1.45	1.55
8%	1.35	1.45
10%	1.25	1.35
12%	1.15	1.25
14%	1.05	1.15
16%	1.0	1.05
18%	0.9	0.95
20%	0.8	0.85

Source: based on Gibbs, Householder, and Potter (1996).

How to calculate the amount of a specific nutrient contained in a feed

Use one of the following general rules to determine the amount of a nutrient in a feed according to whether one is using an as sampled basis or a dry matter basis:

1. *Dry matter basis:* Multiply the amount of feed, dry matter basis, by the % nutrient on a dry matter basis.
2. *As sampled basis:* Multiply the amount of feed, as sampled basis, by the % nutrient on an as sampled basis.

Example:

You are feeding 20 pounds (as sampled) of first cutting hay to your horse. The forage analysis indicates the following nutrient content of the hay. Determine the amount of digestible energy and crude protein in the hay using both methods described above:

	As Sampled	**Dry Matter**
DM	91%	100%
DE	0.79 Mcal/lb	0.87 Mcal/lb
CP	8.2%	9.0%

Method 1: Dry matter basis

1. It would first be necessary to convert the amount as sampled to the corresponding amount of dry matter:

    $20\,lb \times 0.91 = 18.2\,lb$ dry matter

2. Then determine the DE and crude protein using the analyses from the dry matter basis:

    DE : $18.2\,lb$ dry matter $\times 0.87\,Mcal/lb = 15.8\,Mcal\,DE$

    CP : $18.2\,lb$ dry matter $\times 0.09 = 1.64\,lb\,CP$

Method 2: As sampled basis

Since the forage analysis provides nutrient percentages on as an sampled basis, it's not necessary to calculate the dry matter first.

1. Multiply the amount as sampled by DE and % CP on as sampled basis:

    DE : $20\,lb \times 0.79\,Mcal/lb = 15.8\,Mcal\,DE$

    CP : $20\,lb \times 0.082 = 1.64\,lb\,CP$

Note: Some tables only report nutrient percentages on a dry matter basis, making Method 1 the format to use in those situations.

The conventional method for rounding answers to the nearest hundredth's place is to look at the number in the thousandth's place. If that number is between 0 and 4, the number in the hundredth's place remains as is; if the thousandth's place digit is 5 or greater, then the hundredth's number is rounded up.

For example, the following numbers rounded to the hundredth's place are as follows:

3.144   rounds to   3.14

3.145   rounds to   3.15

3.197   rounds to   3.20

Compare the answers from Method 1 to Method 2. They are the same!

NOTES:

Practice problems: Calculating the amount of nutrients in feeds

1. The analysis of the nutrients from a grass hay is shown below. (These percentages would have been obtained from a forage analysis.) Determine the amounts of each nutrient listed below that would be provided by 25 pounds of the hay fed on an as sampled basis. <u>Show your work for both methods.</u>

	As Sampled Basis	Dry Matter Basis
DM	90%	100%
DE	0.82 Mcal/lb	0.91 Mcal/lb
CP	9.54%	10.6%
Ca	0.54%	0.6%
P	0.126%	0.14%

a. Amount of digestible energy (DE):
    Method 1:

    Method 2:

b. Amount of crude protein (CP):
    Method 1:

    Method 2:

c. Amount of calcium (Ca):
    Method 1:

    Method 2:

d. Amount of phosphorus (P):
    Method 1:

    Method 2:

2. A mature working horse is fed 8 pounds of Scholar Horse Feed (introduced in Lab 5) per day. Several of the nutrients from the guaranteed analysis are listed below. Recall that the nutrient composition of commercial feeds is reported on an as sampled basis (review sidebar, page 93). Determine the amount of each nutrient listed below provided by the 8 pounds of Scholar Horse Feed. Remember to label the units of each nutrient.

Scholar Horse Feed, guaranteed analysis:

Crude protein (min.)	13.0%
Crude fat (min.)	6.0%
Crude fiber (max.)	8.0%
Calcium (min.)	1.0%
Phosphorus (min.)	0.85%

a. Digestible energy (consult Table 7.1 to determine the DE of the Scholar Horse Feed)

b. Crude protein

c. Calcium

d. Phosphorus

Reference:

Gibbs, P., Householder, D., Potter, G. (1996). *Selection and Use of Feedstuffs in Horse Feeding.* M. Benefield (Ed.). Retrieved from Texas A&M University Department of Animal Science: https://animalscience.tamu.edu/wp-content/uploads/sites/14/2012/04/nutrition-selection-and-use-of-roughage-in-horses.pdf.

Supplemental Activity
TRIP TO THE FEED STORE

Materials:

- Feed store

Objective:

The purpose of this activity is to have students look at the nutrition information displayed on various feed products and supplements.

Activity:

1. Travel to your local feed provider.

2. Locate the nutrition information on bags of grain, salt blocks, and other supplements. If the store sells hay, ask for a forage analysis.

3. Answer the following questions:

    a. Was the information easy to find and/or readily available?

    b. What steps, if any, could feed companies or stores make to help customers match the right feed to their horse's needs?

    c. For your own horse, which feeds and supplements would you use and why?

Name_____

Lab Section_____

Lab 7 Assignment

DETERMINING SPECIFIC NUTRIENTS WITHIN A FEED

1. A forage analysis of a mixed grass hay reported the following nutrients:

	As Sampled Basis	**Dry Matter Basis**
DM	91%	100%
DE	0.73 Mcal/lb	0.80 Mcal/lb
CP	7.9%	8.7%

You are feeding 25 pounds (as sampled) of this hay per day. Determine the amounts of digestible energy and crude protein in the hay using Method 1 (dry matter basis) and Method 2 (as sampled basis).

a. Digestible energy:
    Method 1 (dry matter basis):

    Method 2 (as sampled basis):

b. Crude protein:
    Method 1 (dry matter basis):

    Method 2 (as sampled basis):

2. You are feeding your horse 5 pounds of rolled oats (as sampled basis) daily. According to the NRC, 2007 (pp. 304), the nutrient content for DE and CP of the rolled oats is listed below (Please note that the DE has been changed from Mcal/kg to Mcal/lb. This will be further explored in Lab 8.)

    DM (% As Sampled)   90.0%

    DE (DM basis)   1.49 Mcal/lb

    CP (DM basis)   13.2%

    Calculate the amount of digestible energy and crude protein that the horse is receiving from the rolled oats. Remember that the percentages provided by the NRC are only on a dry matter basis. Please show your work.

    a. Digestible energy:

    b. Crude protein

3. A horse is fed 28 pounds of mixed grass hay and 6 pounds of commercial pellets each day. The nutrient composition for both the hay and grain are listed below. Using Method 2 (as sampled basis), please determine the amount of each nutrient listed below. Use the space provided to show your calculations and label all units. Place your answers in the blanks provided.

| | Mixed Grass Hay | | Commercial Pellets |
	As Sampled Basis	Dry Matter Basis	As Sampled Basis
DM	90%	100%	90%
DE	0.81 Mcal/lb	0.9 Mcal/lb	_____ (Consult Table 7.1)
CP	7.7%	8.5%	12%
Crude fat	Not reported	Not reported	5%
Crude fiber	Not reported	Not reported	10%
Ca	0.6%	0.66%	1.25%
P	0.26%	0.29%	0.55%

    a. Determine the amount of digestible energy from the hay: _____

    b. Determine the amount of digestible energy from the pellets: _____
        (note: Table 7.1 will need to be consulted for this)

    c. Determine the total amount of DE: _____

d. Determine the amount of crude protein from the hay: _____

e. Determine the amount of crude protein from the pellets: _____

f. Determine the total amount of crude protein: _____

g. Determine the amount of calcium from the hay: _____

h. Determine the amount of calcium from the pellets: _____

i. Determine the total amount of calcium: _____

j. Determine the amount of phosphorus from the hay: _____

k. Determine the amount of phosphorus from the pellets: _____

l. Determine the total amount of phosphorus: _____

Challenge questions:

1. Give a brief description of the relationship between *crude fiber* and *digestible energy*. Then tell what happens to *digestible energy* when **crude fat** increases in the diet.

2. Using a forage analysis that is provided, determine the amount of DM, DE, CP, Ca, and P that an assigned horse receives daily from its forage. Please show all calculations.

Laboratory 8
THE USE OF FEEDING STANDARDS
AND ENGLISH-METRIC CONVERSIONS

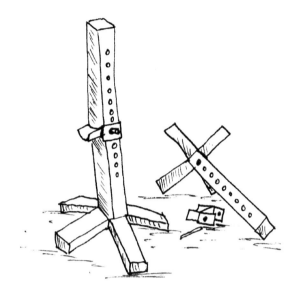

Source: Rachel Monticelli-Turner.

Introduction:

One purpose of this laboratory exercise is to assist the student in determining specific nutrient requirements and total intake needs of different types of horses. This will be done through the use of tables called feeding standards. A second purpose of this lab is to remind students about differences between the U.S. system of measures, called the English system of measurement, and the more universal system of measures, called the metric system.

Objectives:

When finished with the material from this lab, the student should be able to:

1. Determine the requirements for digestible energy (DE), crude protein (CP), calcium (Ca), phosphorus (P) and Vitamin A for horses of various weights, ages, and athletic demands.

2. Determine the daily potential intake for horses of various weights, ages, and athletic demands.

3. Convert units back and forth from the English system of measurement to the metric system.

Question for further discussion:

1. What environmental factors could positively or negatively affect a horse's daily nutrient requirements?

Manual of Equine Nutrition and Feeding Management, First Edition.
Carol Z. Buckhout and Barbara E. Lindberg.
© 2022 John Wiley & Sons, Inc. Published 2022 by John Wiley & Sons, Inc.
Companion website: www.wiley.com/go/buckhout/manual

General overview

Equine nutritionists have spent a great deal of time determining nutrient requirements of various classes of horses. The results of their work can be found in tables that are collectively called feeding standards. Such tables can be found in the National Research Council *Nutrient Requirements of Horses* (2007) beginning with Table 16-1 found on page 294. This set of tables serves as the basis for diet formulation for all classes of horses.

Feeding standards serve as guidelines to assist with ration formulation. Each animal is an individual and may have slightly different needs based on such factors as:

- Size
- Age
- Period of growth
- Amount of exercise
- Gestation stage
- Lactation
- Other factors such as health status, stress, etc.

While there are many nutrients essential for optimum health and performance, generally five (5) basic categories are considered when balancing a ration (Lewis, 1996):

1. *Energy:* reported as digestible energy (DE) and measured in units of calories (cal) or megacalories (Mcal) 1 Mcal = 1,000,000 calories; previously, energy was reported as Total Digestible Nutrients (TDN).

2. *Protein:* reported as either crude protein (CP) or digestible protein (DP) and measured in units of pounds (lb), ounces (oz) or grams (g). Since lysine (lys) is such an important limiting amino acid, it may be listed separately.

3. *Minerals:* calcium and phosphorus are two common macro minerals to evaluate in an equine diet. They are measured in grams or ounces. Important micro minerals such as selenium, iron, copper and zinc are measured in parts per million (ppm).

4. *Vitamins:* Vitamin A is often evaluated and it may also be necessary to monitor Vitamin E; vitamins are measured in International Units (IU).

5. *Daily feed intake:* a function of the horse's body weight, level of activity and individual needs; most horses consume between 2% and 2.5% of their body weight in total feed per day; most feeding standard tables provide suggestions for daily intake.

International Units (IU):

This unit of measure is used primarily for vitamins A, D, and E and sometimes for medications. It is based on potency, not on a volume or a weight. Different vitamins and medications have different potencies which affects their requirements as well as their conversions to units such as milligrams. Therefore, there is no standard equivalent between International Units and milligrams.

Mineral ratios

The relative amounts of minerals in the equine diet are important to consider for proper growth and metabolism. For example: the ideal ratio of calcium to phosphorus is 1.5:1 and the best ratio of zinc to copper is 3:1 or 4:1. Excessive levels of iron can affect the utilization of minerals such as copper. The optimal ratio iron to copper to zinc is 4:1:3.

English/metric conversions:

Since nutrition is an international subject, it is necessary to review how the U.S. system of measures (sometimes called English units or U.S. customary units) compares to the metric system. Review the conversions between the English and metric systems listed below and apply them to the appropriate examples and assignment problems included in this lab.

1 kg	=	2.204 lb
1 lb	=	0.4536 kg
453.6 g	=	1 lb
1 kg	=	1000 g
1 g	=	1000 mg
1 oz	=	28.35 g
1 g	=	0.053 oz
1 metric ton	=	2204.6 lb

Units given	Conversion	Units Obtained
kg	× 2.2	lb
lb	÷ 2.2	kg
kg	× 1000	g
g	÷ 1000	kg
g	÷ 453.6	lb
lb	× 453.6	g
g	÷ 28.35	oz
oz	× 28.35	g
Mcal/kg	÷ 2.2	Mcal/lb
Mcal/lb	× 2.2	Mcal/kg
mg/kg	=	ppm
ppm	× 0.4536	mg/lb

Abbreviations:

g = gram

kg = kilogram

mg = milligram

lb = pound

oz = ounce

ppm = parts per million

English Units Reminders

1 lb = 16 oz

1 English ton = 2000 lb

Calorie Units:

c = calorie

Kcal = kilocalorie

Mcal = megacalorie

1 Kcal = 1,000 c

1 Mcal = 1,000,000 c

1,000 Kcal = 1 Mcal

Laboratory 8 Examples And Activity
USING FEEDING STANDARDS TO DETERMINE NUTRIENT REQUIREMENTS FOR DIFFERENT CLASSES OF HORSES

Reference: Tables 16-3 and 16-4, pp. 298–301, provided in NRC (2007) Nutrient Requirements of Horses, Sixth Edition.

When determining nutrient requirements for the following animals please **LABEL ALL UNITS!!!**

EXAMPLE 1:

Determine the nutrient requirements of a 500 kg average maintenance horse.

Solution: Use NRC (2007) Table 16-3 (page 298) to determine DE, CP, Ca, P, and Vitamin A. Consult the footnotes for the percentage of body weight to use in determining total feed intake.

DE	CP	Ca	P	Vit. A
16.7 Mcal	630 g	20 g	14 g	15 (10³) IU

Percentage of body weight recommended: <u>2%</u> (see footnotes) current body weight: <u>500 kg</u>

Daily feed intake: 0.02 × 500 = 10 kg or 10 kg × 2.2 lb/kg = 22 lb feed

EXAMPLE 2:

Determine the nutrient requirements of a 500 kg working horse, which is exercised at a moderate level of exercise.

Solution: Use NRC (2007) Table 16-3 (page 298) to determine DE, CP, Ca, P, and Vitamin A. Consult the footnotes for the percentage of body weight to use in determining total feed intake.

DE	CP	Ca	P	Vit. A
_____ Mcal	_____ g	_____ g	_____ g	_____ IU

Percentage of body weight recommended: _____   Current body weight: _____

kg of daily feed intake: _____

lb of daily feed intake: _____

EXAMPLE 3:

Determine the nutrient requirements of a yearling horse with an estimated mature body weight of 600 kg.

Solution: Use NRC (2007) Table 16-4 (page 300) to determine DE, CP, Ca, P, and Vitamin A. Consult the footnotes for the percentage of body weight to use in determining total feed intake. Remember that a yearling is not full grown, so carefully observe the table for its current body weight.

DE	CP	Ca	P	Vit. A
_____ Mcal	_____ g	_____ g	_____ g	_____ IU

Percentage of body weight recommended: _____   Current body weight: _____

kg of daily feed intake: _____

lb of daily feed intake: _____

Supplemental Activity
THE NRC COMPUTER PROGRAM

Materials:

- Computer
- Internet connection

Objective:

The objective of this activity is to introduce students to the resources of the free NRC computer program.

1. Go to the following website: http://nrc88.nas.edu/nrh .

2. A gray pop-up box will appear. You will need to click OK in order to use the program.

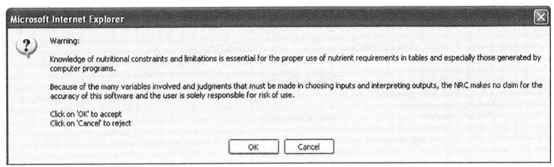

Source: Microsoft Corporation

3. Click on "Animal Specification" to reveal that part of the program.

4. Use information from the questions in this lab's activities or assignment. The line labeled "Animal Requirements" will change as information is changed in the "Animal Specification" section of the program.

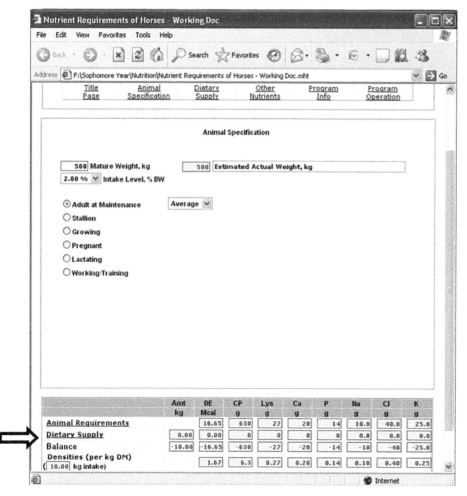

Source: Microsoft Corporation

Tip: In Internet Explorer click on "File" and then "Save As". This will allow you to save the computer program to your computer, so that you will not need an internet connection every time you use it.

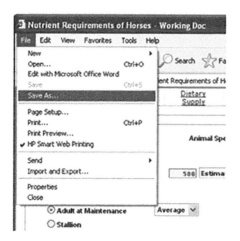

Source: Microsoft Corporation

Supplemental activity continued:

Using the Animal Specification portion of the NRC computer program; determine the nutrient requirements for the following types of horses.

1. 500 kg mature weight; high maintenance

DE	CP	Ca	P
_____	_____	_____	_____

2. 700 kg mature weight
    Growing horse; 5 months of age
    Estimated actual weight, kg _____

DE	CP	Lys	Ca	P
_____	_____	_____	_____	_____

3. 650 kg mature weight
    Working/training horse; heavy work load

DE	CP	Ca	P
_____	_____	_____	_____

4. 525 kg mature weight pregnant mare; 8 months of gestation
    Estimated actual weight _____

DE	CP	Ca	P
_____	_____	_____	_____

Metric Conversion Problems

1.   4 kg =   _____ g

2.   800 g =   _____ kg

3.   15 kg =   _____ g

4.   9000 g =   _____ kg

5.   50 g =   _____ mg

6.   10 kg =   _____ lb

7.   500 kg =   _____ lb

8.   100 lb =   _____ kg

9.   1200 lb =   _____ kg

10.   40 lb =   _____ g

11.   32 g =   _____ kg

12.   300 g =   _____ lb

13.   3 Mcal/kg =   _____ Mcal/lb

14.   1.4 Mcal/lb =   _____ Mcal/kg

15.   1100 Kcal/lb =   _____ Mcal/lb

References:

Lewis, L. (1996). *Feeding and Care of the Horse* (2nd ed.). Media, PA: Lippincott, Williams and Wilkens.

National Research Council. (2007). *Nutrient Requirements of Horses* (6th ed.). Washington: The National Academies Press.

Name _____

Lab Section __ _____

Laboratory 8 Assignment
DETERMINING NUTRIENT REQUIREMENTS

Determine the nutrient requirements for the following animals and please LABEL ALL UNITS!! (ex: Mcal, g, oz, %) Reference: NRC (2007)

1. **A 600 kg working horse exercised at moderate work:**

   DE   CP   Ca   P   Vit. A

   _____   _____   _____   _____   _____

   Percentage of its body weight recommended?: _____

   kg of daily feed intake: _____

   lb of daily feed intake: _____

2. **A 24-month-old growing horse, that is estimated to mature at 400 kg, exercised at light exercise:**

   DE   CP   Ca   P   Vit. A

   _____   _____   _____   _____   _____

   Percentage of its body weight recommended?: _____   Current body weight?: _____

   kg of daily feed intake: _____

   lb of daily feed intake: _____

3. **A 500 kg pregnant mare in her 10th month of gestation:**

    DE   CP   Ca   P   Vit. A

    _____   _____   _____   _____   _____

    Percentage of its body weight recommended?: _____ Current body weight?: _____

    kg of daily feed intake: _____

    lb of daily feed intake: _____

4. **An 880 pound lactating mare in her first month of lactation:**

    DE   CP   Ca   P   Vit. A

    _____   _____   _____   _____   _____

    Percentage of its body weight recommended?: _____   Current body weight?: _____

    kg of daily feed intake: _____

    lb of daily feed intake: _____

Metric/English Conversions:

1. 600 g = _____ kg

2. 25 lb = _____ kg

3. 18 kg = _____ lb

4. 3.4 kg = _____ g

5. 300 g = _____ lb

6. 500 g = _____ kg

7. 3 lb = _____ g

8. 2439 lb = _____ kg

9. 28 g = _____ lb

10. 2.5 Mcal/kg = _____ Mcal/lb

11. 0.9 Mcal/lb = _____ Mcal/kg

12. 1850 kcal/lb = _____ Mcal/lb

13. 1.35 Mcal/kg = _____ kcal/kg

14. 24 lb alfalfa hay = _____ kg of alfalfa hay

15. 15 kg corn = _____ lb of corn

16. 0.35 lb of salt = _____ g of salt

17. 1 T (English) of grass hay = _____ kg of grass hay

18. 5000 g soybean meal = _____ lb of soybean meal

19. 3.5 ounces (oz) of calcium = _____ g of calcium

20. A 550 kg horse weighs _____ lb

NOTES:

Laboratory 9
RATION EVALUATION PART I

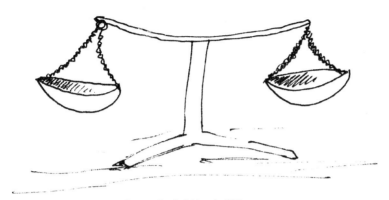

Source: Rachel Monticelli-Turner.

Introduction:

The purpose of this laboratory exercise is to instruct students about how to evaluate the diet of a horse. The goal is to determine whether a horse's daily nutrient requirements are being met. This process will require the application of knowledge learned in all previous labs, especially Labs 7 and 8.

Objectives:

When finished with the material from this lab the student should be able to:

1. Compare the nutrient requirements of a specific horse to the amount of nutrients that it receives through its feed.
2. Make recommendations for potential changes in a horse's diet.

Questions for further discussion:

1. When observing the results from evaluating rations:
   a. Is there a nutrient that is consistently in excess of a horse's requirements? If so, how can one adjust the horse's diet?
   b. Is there a nutrient that is consistently a deficit as compared to a horse's requirements? What recommendations would you make to adjust for this?

Manual of Equine Nutrition and Feeding Management, First Edition.
Carol Z. Buckhout and Barbara E. Lindberg.
© 2022 John Wiley & Sons, Inc. Published 2022 by John Wiley & Sons, Inc.
Companion website: www.wiley.com/go/buckhout/manual

NOTES:

Analysis vs. Evaluation

The true definition of analysis refers to the chemical analysis of a feedstuff. However, it is common to informally use the word "analysis" to also mean "evaluation" when referring to the examination of all the components of a ration.

Introduction to Ration Evaluation

If one knows the nutrient requirements of a horse based on its body weight, stage of growth and/or activity level, (covered in Lab 8), it is possible to evaluate whether its requirements are being met from a current diet. Information about the nutrient content of the feeds being used is needed in this process. From previous labs, we have learned that laboratory analyses of forages being fed are most accurate. However in the situation where a forage analysis is not available, feed composition tables are also very useful. We have also learned that all purchased grain mixes must come labeled with a guaranteed analysis that provides information about the crude protein, crude fat, and crude fiber content. It's quite possible that additional information about the nutrient content of the mix is also included on the feed label. When individual grains are fed to horses, one may rely on feed composition tables to provide the nutrient content of a particular grain. A good example in this case would be oats, because they continue to be a popular cereal grain to feed to horses. In all cases, one needs to know the weight of forages or concentrate being fed and the nutrient content of the forage(s) and grain(s) in order to determine the specific amount of nutrients that the horse is receiving from its feeds.

A note about feed composition tables: notice whether the nutrient content is reported on a dry matter basis or on an as sampled basis, or both. Table 6, page 419 in Lewis (1996) and Table 16-6, pages 304–307 in NRC (2007) both report nutrient composition on a dry matter basis. Forage analyses usually report nutrient composition on both a dry matter and an as sampled basis. Feed labels from commercial grain mixes report nutrient composition on an as sampled basis. Keeping track of which basis (dry matter or as sampled) becomes important when doing a ration analysis.

Example 1: A 500 kg average maintenance horse is being fed a diet of 10 kg (22 lb) of mature, cool season grass hay (10 kg or 22 lb is 2% of the horse's body weight). The animal is getting no additional grain in its diet. Consult Tables 16-3 and 16-6 in NRC (2007). Analyze whether the hay alone meets the horse's nutrient requirements for total intake, DE, CP, Ca, and P:

> ***Step 1:*** To determine the nutrient content of the grass hay cool season, mature; consult NRC (2007) Table 16-6, pp. 306; all nutrients are listed on a dry matter basis:

DM:	84.4%
DE:	2.04 Mcal/kg = 0.93 Mcal/lb
CP:	10.8%
Ca:	0.47%
P:	0.26%

Remember, the terms "as sampled" and "as fed" may be used interchangeably.

<u>Note:</u>

$$\frac{Mcal}{kg} \div \frac{2.2\,kg}{lb} = \frac{Mcal}{lb}$$

Step 2: Determine the amount of nutrients in 10 kg or 22 lb of the grass hay.

$$DM: 22 \, lb \times 0.844 = 18.6 \, lb \, DM$$

$$DE: 18.6 \, lb \, DM \times 0.93 \, Mcal \, / \, lb = 17.3 \, Mcal$$

$$CP: 18.6 \, lb \, DM \times 0.108 = 2 \, lb \, CP$$

$$2 \, lb \times 453.6 \, g \, / \, lb = 907 \, g \, CP$$

$$Ca: 18.6 \, lb \, DM \times 0.0047 = 0.087 \, lb \, Ca$$

$$0.087 \, lb \times 453.6 \, g \, / \, lb = 39.5 \, g \, Ca$$

$$P: 18.6 \, lb \, DM \times 0.0026 = 0.048 \, lb \, P$$

$$0.048 \, lb \, P \times 453.6 \, g \, / \, lb = 21.8 \, g$$

Step 3: Determine the horse's nutrient requirements for DE, CP, Ca, and P by Consulting Table 16-3 page 298 of the NRC (2007). Is there a positive or negative difference between the provided and the required amounts?

	DE (Mcal)	CP (g)	Ca (g)	P (g)
Provided (*step 2*):	17.3	907	39.5	21.8
Required (*step 3*):	16.7	630	20.0	14.0
Difference (+/−):	+0.6	+277	+19.5	+7.8

According to this evaluation, are the nutrient requirements of the 500 kg average maintenance horse being met? _____

Example 2: Evaluate a ration for a 500 kg working horse exercised at a moderate level. The horse is fed according to NRC guidelines of 2.25% of its body weight per day. It receives a combination of 5 pounds of rolled oats and the rest of its intake is a mostly grass hay, mid-mature. Use information provided by Tables 16-3 and 16-6 in the NRC (2007) to evaluate whether the animal's nutrient requirements are met. Note that 2.25% of the horse's body weight = 24.75 lb per day. To accommodate for potential loss or waste of feed, 24.75 pounds may be rounded up to 25 lb.

Step 1: Nutrient content of the mostly grass hay, mid-mature:
(NRC (2007) Table 16-6, pp. 306)

DM:	87.3%
DE:	2.19 Mcal/kg = 1.0 Mcal/lb (rounded up)
CP:	17.4%
Ca:	0.88%
P:	0.36%

Nutrient content of rolled oats: (NRC (2007) Table 16-6, pp. 304)

DM:	90%
DE:	3.27 Mcal/kg = 1.48 Mcal/lb
CP:	13.2%
Ca:	0.11%
P:	0.40%

Step 2: Set up a chart to calculate the nutrients provided in the feeds.

Step 3: Consult the correct NRC (2007) table for the horse's requirements and record these in the appropriate category. Compare nutrient totals to requirements.

Feed	As Fed	DM		DE		CP		Ca		P	
	lb	%	lb	Mcal/lb	Mcal	%	lb	%	lb	%	lb
Hay	20	87.3		1.00		17.4		0.88		0.36	
Oats	5	90.0		1.48		13.2		0.11		0.40	
Total	25										
Convert to g*							g		g		g
Required:							g		g		g
Difference (+/−):							g		g		g

*Pounds of CP, Ca, and P must be converted to grams to compare to the horse's requirements

According to your evaluation, are the nutrient requirements of this working horse being met? _____

References:

Lewis, L. (1996). *Feeding and Care of the Horse* (2nd ed.). Media, PA: Lippincott, Williams and Wilkens.

National Research Council. (2007). *Nutrient Requirements of Horses* (6th ed.). Washington: The National Academies Press.

Supplemental Activity
EXCEL SHEET

Materials:

- Computer with Microsoft Excel
- Nutrient requirements for particular horse
- Feed label and forage analysis or feed composition tables

Objective:

The purpose of this activity is to introduce students to how a computer program, such as Microsoft Excel, can make performing ration evaluation easier.

Activity:

1. Open a new Microsoft Excel document.
2. Create a chart similar to the one below.

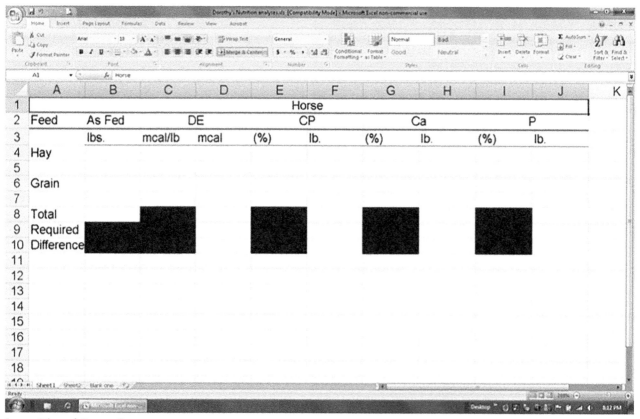

Source: Microsoft Corporation

3. Next enter the known values, such as the amount of hay and the percentages available of the different nutrients.

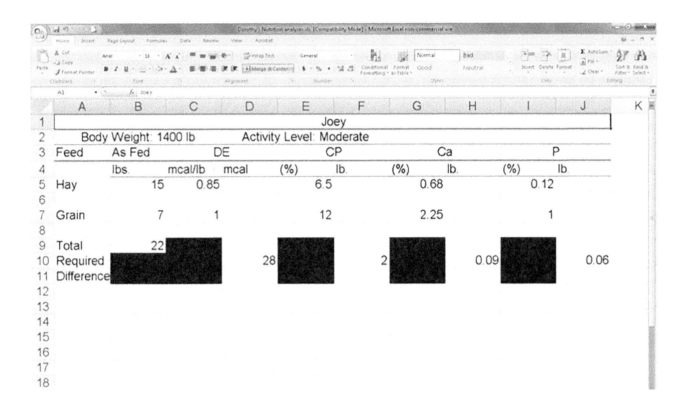

Source: Microsoft Corporation

4. To fill in the missing cells write the appropriate formulas in the cell. To write a formula start with the "=" sign. Then click on the cell (or type the cell's designation, for example A1) that the arithmetic function will be applied to. Next, choose the correct arithmetic function (type a × for multiplication, a + for addition, etc). Then click on or type the cell designation of the second cell.

Examples:

To multiply two cells:= B5 × C5

To add two cells: = D5 + D7

To subtract two cells: D9 − D10

For other arithmetic functions consult the functions bar in Excel, which is denoted by the fx symbol.

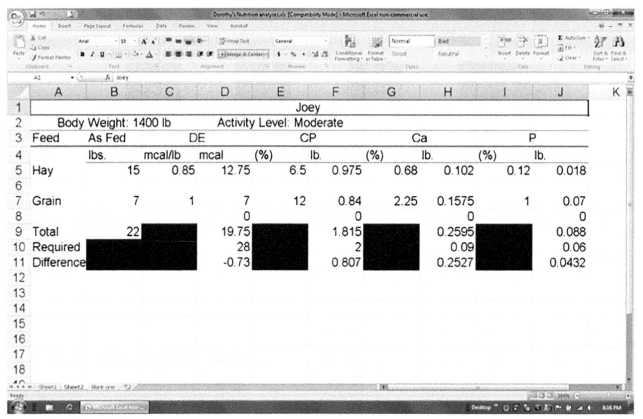

Source: Microsoft Corporation

5. Now if you decide to increase or decrease the amount of hay or grain fed, simply change the amount in the as fed column and the totals and differences will change accordingly.

This Supplemental Activity is based on a Microsoft Excel chart a Microsoft Excel chart created by Dorothy Robertson, Cazenovia College '09.

Name_____

Lab Section_____

Laboratory 9 Assignment
RATION EVALUATION

1. Evaluate a ration for a mature working horse, weighing 600 kg, exercised at the moderate work level. The horse is currently being fed at the NRC (2007) recommended level of 2.25% of its body weight per day. It receives 8 pounds of rolled oats daily and the rest of its intake is in grass hay, cool season, mid-mature. Using the format established in the examples, evaluate whether this horse's nutrient requirements for DE, CP, Ca, and P are satisfied. Use information from tables of Nutrient Composition and Daily Nutrient Requirements from NRC (2007) to complete this analysis.

Horse's Body Weight _____lb

2.25% of the Horse's Body Weight _____lb

Feed	As Fed	DM		DE		CP		Ca		P	
	lb	%	lb	Mcal/lb*	Mcal	%	lb	%	lb	%	lb
Hay											
Grain											
Total											
Convert to g								g		g		g
Required:							g		g		g
Difference (+/−):							g		g		g

Since DE is listed as Mcal/kg in the NRC tables, be sure to convert it to Mcal/lb.

Are the horse's nutrient requirements met? _____

2. A 500 kg pregnant mare in her 10th month of gestation is being fed at the NRC (2007) recommended level of 2% of her <u>current</u> body weight. She receives a mixed grass and legume hay, mid-mature, and 6 pounds of rolled oats. Evaluate whether the mare's nutrient requirements are satisfied. Use information from tables of Nutrient Composition and Daily Nutrient Requirements from NRC (2007) to complete this evaluation.

Mare's Current Body Weight _____lb

2% of Mare's Current Body Weight _____lb

Feed	As Fed	DM		DE		CP		Ca		P	
	lb	%	lb	Mcal/lb*	Mcal	%	lb	%	lb	%	lb
Hay											
Grain											
Total											
Convert to g							g		g		g
Required:							g		g		g
Difference (+/−):							g		g		g

*Since DE is listed as Mcal/kg in the NRC tables, be sure to convert it to Mcal/lb.

Are the mare's nutrient requirements met?_____

Laboratory 10
RATION EVALUATION PART II

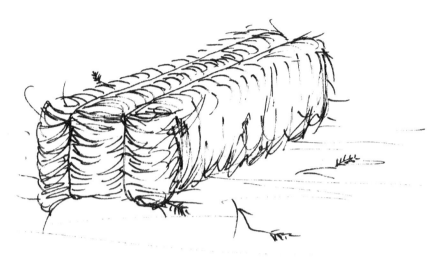

Source: Rachel Monticelli-Turner.

Introduction:

The purpose of this laboratory exercise is to enable the student to evaluate a horse's ration using information from a commercial feed label and from a forage analysis.

Objectives:

When finished with this exercise, the student should be able to:

1. Correctly interpret information provided on a feed label in order to evaluate a ration.
2. Evaluate horse rations using current information.
3. Make appropriate recommendations for horse rations.

Question for further discussion:

1. Why should feed store managers be interested in forage analyses for their clients?

Manual of Equine Nutrition and Feeding Management, First Edition.
Carol Z. Buckhout and Barbara E. Lindberg.
© 2022 John Wiley & Sons, Inc. Published 2022 by John Wiley & Sons, Inc.
Companion website: www.wiley.com/go/buckhout/manual

NOTES:

NOTES:

Introduction:
Utilizing the information on a commercial feed label

There are several categories of information that must be provided on a commercial feed label according to the standards set by the Uniform State Feed Bill (Briggs, 2001). The bill was adopted in 1994 by the Association of American Feed Control Officials (AAFCO) in order to standardize the types of information that should be provided to purchasers. A brief summary of the categories is below (Briggs, 2001).

1. Product name, purpose and a brief description of its format (pellet, sweet feed, etc.).

2. The *guaranteed analysis* of feed ingredients. At the very minimum, the following nutrients should be listed:
    a. Crude protein: listed as a minimum percent
    b. Crude fat: listed as a minimum percent
    c. Crude fiber: listed as a maximum percent
    d. Calcium: minimum and maximum percentages listed
    e. Phosphorus: minimum percentage listed
    f. Copper: listed as parts per million (ppm)
    g. Zinc: listed as parts per million (ppm)
    h. Selenium: listed as parts per million (ppm)
    i. Vitamin A: listed as International Units (IU) per pound

3. Ingredients list: Manufacturers are allowed by the AAFCO to list feed ingredients in general terms such as processed grain by-products or "plant protein products" as opposed to specific feeds like soybean meal, corn gluten feed, or wheat bran. This flexibility makes it possible for the actual combination of feeds to change slightly as their prices change. However, the overall nutritional content of the commercial feed cannot change according to the *guaranteed analysis*. This rule is controlled on a state by state basis. Florida actually requires as specific listing of the feed ingredients provided (Briggs, 2001).

4. Feeding instructions: These would be based on the body weight of the horse, its age, and its activity level.

A challenge for ration evaluation when using commercial feeds is that the digestible energy (DE) is not included on the feed label. However, both crude fat and crude fiber are indicators of the energy content. Tables, such as Table 7.1 provided in Lab 7 and again on the next page, are available that equate DE to crude fat and crude fiber levels. While the values on the chart may not be exact for every commercial feed, one can extrapolate to determine a fairly accurate DE content of a specific feed.

Examples of determining DE based on crude fat and crude fiber: (see Table 10.1, below)

1. Crude fat: 3%
    Crude fiber: 12%
    Based on the above values the DE would be 1.15 Mcal/lb.

2. Crude fat: 6%
    Crude fiber: 8%
    Based on the above values, the DE would be 1.45 Mcal/lb.

3. Crude fat: 7%
    Crude fiber: 15%
    One can extrapolate from the chart that DE would be
        1.10 Mcal/lb.

Table 10.1
Correlations Between Crude Fiber,
Crude Fat, and Digestible Energy

Crude Fiber	DE, Mcal/lb (≤5% Crude Fat)	DE, Mcal/lb (>5% Crude Fat)
2%	1.65	1.75
4%	1.55	1.65
6%	1.45	1.55
8%	1.35	1.45
10%	1.25	1.35
12%	1.15	1.25
14%	1.05	1.15
16%	1.0	1.05
18%	0.9	0.95
20%	0.8	0.85

Source: Gibbs, Householder, and Potter (1996).

NOTES:

Example Ration Evaluation Using a Forage Analysis and a Commercial Feed Label:

A 600 kg horse used in a lesson program is worked weekly at a moderate level. It receives a daily ration of mixed grass hay and a commercial concentrate called Scholar Horse Feed. The specific amount of hay and grain that the horse is fed is shown below:

Mixed grass hay: 7 flakes/day; an average flake weighs 3.5 lb

Scholar Horse Feed: 6 pounds per day

Using the format established in Lab 9, evaluate this horse's daily diet for total intake, DE, CP, Ca, and P. A forage analysis of the mixed grass hay is provided below along with the feed label from the Scholar Horse Feed on the following page. Since the forage analysis and the feed label provide the feed nutrients on an as sampled basis, one can ignore the dry matter column when doing the ration analysis. As with Lab 9, the pounds of CP, Ca, and P will need to be converted to grams. However, the DE is already reported in Mcal/lb. Information regarding the horse's daily nutrient requirements may be obtained from the correct chart from the NRC 2007 *Nutrient Requirements of Horses*, sixth revised edition. Use the chart provided on page 142 to complete the evaluation.

SAMPLE FORAGE ANALYSIS: MIXED GRASS HAY

Analyzed for: A Horse Owner

	% Moisture		9.5	
	% Dry matter		90.5	

		As Sampled		Dry Matter
Digestible energy (DE) Mcal/lb		0.89		0.98

	%	g/lb.	%	g/lb.
Crude protein	9.3	42.0	10.2	46.4
Estimated lysine	0.32	1.5	0.36	1.6
Acid Detergent Fiber (ADF)	38.2	173.1	42.2	191.3
Neutral Detergent Fiber (NDF)	63.1	241.0	58.7	266.3
%WSC (Water Sol. Carbs)	7.5	34.2	8.3	37.8
ESC (Simple Sugars)	5.0	22.7	5.5	25.0
Starch	1.4	8.3	1.5	7.0
Non-Fiber Carb (NFC)	19.8	89.8	21.9	99.2

	%	g/lb.	%	g/lb.
Calcium	0.96	4.35	1.06	4.81
Phosphorus	0.18	0.74	0.18	0.82

	As Fed	100% Dry
RFV		89

Scholar Horse Feed

This feed was designed to be fed to the average school horse.

Guaranteed Analysis:

Crude Protein	Min	13.00	%		
Crude Fat	Min	6.00	%		
Crude Fiber	Max	8.00	%		
Calcium	Min	1.00	%	Max	1.20 %
Phosphorus	Min	0.85	%		
Copper	Min	51.00	PPM		
Selenium	Min	0.70	PPM		
Zinc	Min	159.00	PPM		
Vitamin A	Min	3985.30	IU/LB		

Ingredients:

Processed Grain By-Products, Grain Products, Roughage Products, Forage Products, Soybean Meal, Calcium Carbonate, Molasses Products, Plant Protein Products, Salt, Lysine, Methionine Supplement, Natural and Artificial Preservatives, Potassium Chloride, Sodium Selenite, Primaiac, L-Threonine, Zinc Sulfate, Natural & Artificial Flavors added, Copper Sulfate, Selenium Yeast, Selenium, Folic Acid, Zinc Amino Acid Complex, Manganese Supplement, Riboflavin Supplement, Biotin, Thiamine Supplement, Vitamin E Supplement, Vitamin D3 Supplement, Vitamin B12 Supplement, Magnesium Oxide, Cobalt Carbonate, Ferrous Sulfate, Manganese Sulfate, Copper Chloride, Zinc Oxide

***Warning: Do not fed to sheep because it contains supplemental copper.

Product Code: 15638752_THY
Net Wt. 50 LB

Manufactured by:
Scholar Horse Feeds: A Smart Decision
Main Office
Cazenovia, NY, 13035

Lot: 008

Figure 10.1 Feed label example. Source: Sara Tanner Mastellar.

Feed	As Fed	DM		DE		CP		Ca		P	
	lb	%	lb	Mcal/lb	Mcal	%	lb	%	lb	%	lb
Hay**	24.5										
Grain	6.0										
Total											
Convert to g											
Required:											
Difference (+/−):											

* Use Table 10.1 to determine the DE of the Scholar Horse Feed

** Pounds of hay, as fed: 7 flakes/day × 3.5 lb/flake = 24.5 lbs.

Are the horse's nutrient requirements met? _____

Comments:

Supplemental Activity:
APPLYING MICROSOFT EXCEL AND THE NRC COMPUTER PROGRAM

Materials:

- Computer
- Internet connection (if the NRC program is not saved to the computer)
- Excel chart created in the supplemental activity for Lab 8

Objective:

The objective of this activity is to have students utilize the tools of technology to be able to complete ration evaluation more efficiently. Also, this activity will increase the student's amount of experience utilizing the computer programs.

Activity:

1. Use the Excel worksheet created for the supplemental activity for Lab 8 to complete the first question of the assignment for this lab.

2. Use the NRC computer program (see the supplemental activity in Lab 9 for more information) to complete the second question of the assignment for this lab.

   Answer the following questions:

   a. Is it easier for you to do the problems utilizing the computer or by hand with a calculator?

   b. Do you prefer to use the Excel worksheet or the NRC program? Why?

   c. If there are any other ration evaluation programs at your school, how do they compare to the Excel worksheet and the NRC program?

References:

Briggs, K. (2001, October). How to read a feed label. *The Horse*. Retrieved from http://www.thehorse.com/articles/10662/how-to-read-a-feed-label.

Gibbs, P., Householder, D., Potter, G. (1996). *Selection and Use of Feedstuffs in Horse Feeding*. M. Benefield (Ed.). Retrieved from Texas A&M University Department of Animal Science: http://animalscience.tamu.edu/files/2012/04/equine-selection-use-feedstuffs9.pdf.

National Research Council. (2007). *Nutrient Requirements of Horses* (6th ed.). Washington: The National Academies Press.

Name_____

Lab Section_____

Laboratory 10 Assignment

EVALUATING HORSE RATIONS

Evaluate the rations of two assigned horses. It will be necessary to obtain the weights and analyses for all forages and commercial feeds that the horses receive. In addition, it will be necessary to determine the horses' current weights and activity levels.

The chart provided below is enhanced to include more than one type of forage and grain. Items to consider include:

- Current body weight of the horse (pregnant mares and growing horses will weigh differently from their mature body weight).
- Units of measure: Take notice whether you are working with metric or English units.
- As sampled versus dry matter basis: The ration evaluation should be done on an as sampled basis because even though forage analyses may provide both dry matter and as sampled values, feed labels provide as sampled values only.

1. Horse's name: _____   Body weight: _____lb.   _____kg.

   Activity level: _____

Forages Fed	lb	Grains Fed	lb
1 _____	_____	1 _____	_____
2 _____	_____	2 _____	_____
3 _____	_____	3 _____	_____

Feed	As Fed	DM		DE		CP		Ca		P	
	lb	%	lb	Mcal/lb*	Mcal	%	lb	%	lb	%	lb
Hay 1											
Hay 2											
Grain 1											
Grain 2											
Grain 3											
Total											
Convert to g							g		g		g
Required:							g		g		g
Difference (+/−):							g		g		g

*DE values for commercial feeds can be determined using table 10.1

As a final step, calculate the percent body weight fed per day, using the following equation:

$$\frac{lb.feed:\ \rule{2cm}{0.15mm}}{lb.B.W.:\ \rule{2cm}{0.15mm}} = (\rule{1.5cm}{0.15mm})100 = \rule{1.5cm}{0.15mm}\%$$

Comments:

2.   Horse's name: _____   Body weight: _____lb. _____kg.

     Activity level: _____

	Forages Fed		*lb*		*Grains Fed*		*lb*
1	_____		_____	1	_____		_____
2	_____		_____	2	_____		_____
3	_____		_____	3	_____		_____

Feed	*As Fed*	DM		DE		*CP*		*Ca*		*P*	
	lb	%	**lb**	**Mcal/lb***	**Mcal**	**%**	**lb**	**%**	**lb**	**%**	**lb**
Hay 1											
Hay 2											
Grain 1											
Grain 2											
Grain 3											
Total											
Convert to g							g		g		g
Required:							g		g		g
Difference (+/−):							g		g		g

*DE values for commercial feeds can be determined using table 10.1

As a final step, calculate the percent body weight fed per day, using the following equation:

$$\frac{\text{lb.feed:} \quad \rule{2cm}{0.4pt}}{\text{lb.B.W.:} \quad \rule{2cm}{0.4pt}} = (\rule{1.5cm}{0.4pt})\,100 = \rule{1cm}{0.4pt}$$

Comments:

Laboratory 11
THE PEARSON SQUARE

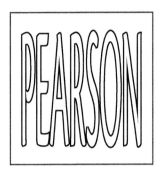

Source: Rachel Monticelli-Turner.

Introduction:

The purpose of this exercise is to instruct students how to formulate a grain mix or a ration that would provide a specific nutrient percentage. This may be done using different feeds, both forages and/or concentrates. The method used is commonly referred to as the Pearson Square.

Objectives:

1. After completing this lab students will be able to utilize the Pearson Square method when formulating a grain ration or an entire ration for a horse.

Questions for further discussion:

1. What are two possible situations that would require a horse to have a ration formulated to meet a specific nutrient percentage?
2. Is it possible to balance a horse's entire daily ration using a series of Pearson Squares?

The Pearson Square

The Pearson Square is a convenient method of formulating feed combinations for a ration, especially grain mix combinations. It can be based on any nutrient, but protein is often a popular target nutrient used with the Pearson Square. Refer to the next page for the steps of the Pearson Square method.

Manual of Equine Nutrition and Feeding Management, First Edition.
Carol Z. Buckhout and Barbara E. Lindberg.
© 2022 John Wiley & Sons, Inc. Published 2022 by John Wiley & Sons, Inc.
Companion website: www.wiley.com/go/buckhout/manual

NOTES:

NOTES:

Procedure for Calculating the Pearson Square:

1. Draw a square and write the desired percentage of nutrient, such as crude protein, in the center. Do not change percentages to their decimal form.

2. Write the nutrient percentage of the lower nutrient, in this case crude protein, by the upper left corner of the square. Then write the percentage of the higher nutrient by the lower left hand corner of the square. The percentage in the center of the square must be less than one corner and greater than the other corner. Again, do not change percentages to their decimal form.

3. Take the positive difference of the upper left corner and the center. Place this number by the lower right-hand corner.

4. Take the positive difference of the lower left corner and the center. Place this number by the upper right-hand corner.

5. The values obtained in steps 3 and 4 represent the ratio of the individual feeds to the total amount. Divide both the upper and lower right-hand corner numbers by their sum. Multiply by 100 and this will calculate the percentages of each feed, as needed in the total mix.

6. Multiply the percentages of each feed by the desired amount of the total mix in order to obtain the specific amounts of each individual feed to add together for the total ration.

Example 1: A feed dealer has been requested to mix a batch of grain to a level of 17% crude protein using corn (analyzed at 9% crude protein) and soybean meal (50% crude protein). In order to make a ton (2000 lb) of this mix, how much of each feed must be used?

Feeds	%CP		Parts	Total Parts		Percent		Total Mix		lb to feed
Corn	9	17	33	÷ 41	=	0.805 or 80.5%	×	2000 lb	=	1610 lb corn
Soybean	50		+8 ——— 41	÷ 41	=	0.195 or 19.5%	×	2000 lb	=	390 lb soybean

Important Points to Remember:

1. One feed ingredient (or combination of feed ingredients) must be lower than the value of the desired mixture (the number in the center of the square) and the other feed ingredient (or combination of feed ingredients) must be higher than the desired mixture.

2. Always subtract diagonally across the square, taking the absolute values between the numbers subtracted (no negative numbers under parts).

3. Even though the subtraction is on the diagonal, the feeds are read horizontally, they do not switch places.

The Pearson Square may also be used with combinations of feeds. In this situation, averages of the nutrient values of the feeds must first be calculated. When the percentages of the feed combinations are determined, divide them according to the proportion that the individual feeds comprise.

Example 2: A feed manufacturer plans to create 500 pounds of a concentrate mix that provides 16% crude protein and with the following feeds available: corn, oats, soybean meal, and corn distillers' grains.

To determine the values on the left hand corners of the square, separate the feeds into low and high protein categories. (This would be the same for any nutrient that is being worked with.)

Feed	Crude Protein % (Lewis, 1996, pp. 419–421)
Corn	9
Oats (regular)	12
Soybean meal	50
Distillers' grains	32

Low protein feeds: corn and oats

Corn provides 9% crude protein, oats provides 12% crude protein; therefore, an average of the low protein feeds is: (9 + 12) ÷ 2 = 10.5%

High protein feeds: soybean meal and corn distillers' grains

Soybean meal provides 50% crude protein and corn distillers' grains provide 32% crude protein, so the average between the two is: (50 + 32) ÷ 2 = 41%.

Feeds	%CP		Parts	Total Parts		Percent		Total Mix		lb to feed
Low protein	10.5		25	÷ 30.5	=	0.820 or 82%	×	500 lb	=	410 lb low protein
High protein	41		+5.5	÷ 30.5	=	0.180 or 18%	×	500 lb	=	90 lb high protein
			30.5							

(center of square = 16)

Determine the pounds of individual feeds:

Low protein:	% in mix		lb		
Corn:	0.50	×	410	=	205 lb
Oats:	0.50	×	410	=	205 lb
Total:				=	410 lb

High protein:	% in mix		lb		
Soybean meal:	0.50	×	90	=	45 lb
Distillers' grain:	0.50	×	90	=	45 lb
Total:				=	90 lb

The Pearson Square may be used to solve for any nutrient that needs to be enhanced in a horse's diet. Further examples may be found in Lewis (1996) pp. 112–137.

References:

Lewis, L. (1996). *Feeding and Care of the Horse* (2nd ed.). Media, PA: Lippincott, Williams and Wilkens.

Supplemental Activity
CREATING A PEARSON SQUARE CALCULATOR IN EXCEL

Materials:

- Computer with Microsoft Excel

Objective:

To have students build a tool in Microsoft Excel that they can utilize for multiple problems.

Activity:

1. Open a new document in Microsoft Excel.
2. Next create the following column headings being sure to leave one blank for the square.
3. To make the square, select the cells you want to be included and put a border around them

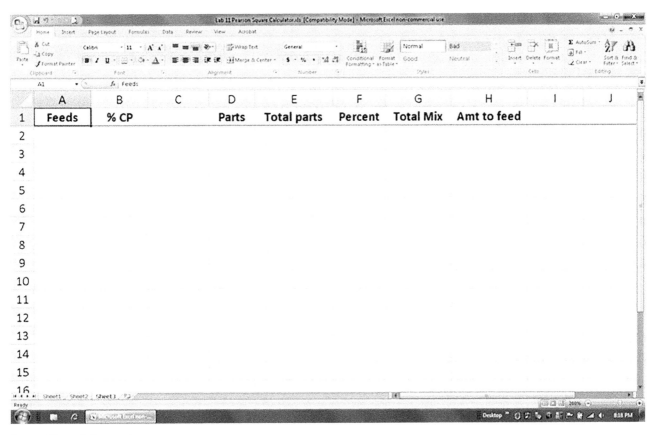

Source: Microsoft Corporation

Tip: If you would like your square to have arrows you can add them by clicking on **insert** and then selecting **shapes**.

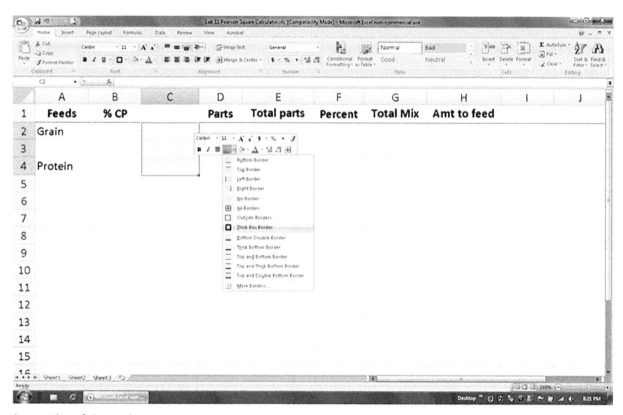

Source: Microsoft Corporation

4. Next add all known values, such as percentages and the amount of the total mix. **Note:** percentages should be entered in decimal form. For example, 8% is equal to 8 divided by 100 or 0.08.

5. Adding formulas is similar to previous supplemental activities. However, the formulas for the right-hand corners of the square are a bit trickier. You will need to use formulas that use absolute value as shown in the next screen shot.

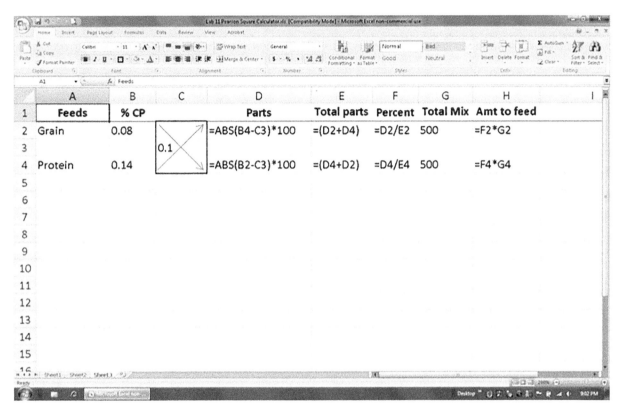

Source: Microsoft Corporation

6. Try your new calculator out on some of the assignment problems.

NOTES:

Name_____

Lab Section_____

Laboratory Assignment 11
PEARSON SQUARE

1. Using the Pearson Square format, formulate a grain mix using oats and soybean meal that when blended provides 13% crude protein. Assume the oats provide 11% crude protein and the soybean meal provides 44% crude protein. The total batch will be 1000 pounds. Determine the pounds of oats and soybean meal that will be needed.

2. Using the Pearson Square format, formulate a grain mix that provides 14% crude protein using the following feeds: corn (9% crude protein), oats (11% crude protein), corn gluten feed (25% crude protein), and soybean meal (44% crude protein). The total batch will be 500 pounds. How many pounds each of corn, oats, corn gluten feed, and soybean meal will be required?

3. Formulate a grain mix that provides 12.5% crude protein using the following feeds: soy hulls (12% crude protein) and ground corn 9% (crude protein), corn distillers' grains (30% crude protein), and soybean meal (48% crude protein). The total batch will be 1 ton. How many pounds each of soy hulls, ground corn, corn distillers' grains, and soybean meal will be required?

4. Use the Pearson Square method to formulate a combination of hay and grain that provides 12% crude protein (as sampled basis). The forage analysis of the hay indicates it provides 11% crude protein, as sampled basis, and the feed label of the grain indicates that the grain provides 14% crude protein. The total amount of hay and grain to feed is 11 kg. Determine the kilograms and pounds of both hay and grain to use.

Challenge Question:

1. Use the Pearson Square method to combine a diet of hay and grain that provides adequate protein for a yearling horse with an estimated mature weight of 500 kg. There are several preliminary steps needed to complete this question:

    a. Determine the total daily intake required.

    b. Determine the percent crude protein needed in the diet of this horse.

    c. When finished with the Pearson Square, use the table provided to determine whether the amounts of hay and grain will provide adequate DE, Ca, and P.

Step 1: *Determine the yearling's total daily intake required.*

The 2007 NRC Table 16-3 (page 298) suggests that the animal be fed 2.5% of its body weight; its current body weight is 321 kg; therefore, daily intake is calculated as follows:

321 kg × 0.025 = _____ kg or _____ lb

Step 2: *Determine the percent protein required by the animal (NRC, 2007 pp. 298).*
First determine this:

Grams CP needed : _____ g or _____ kg

Then calculate this:

Percent protein: $\dfrac{\text{_____ kg protein required}}{\text{_____ kg daily feed}}$ = _____ X 100 = _____ %*

*use this percent in the center of the Pearson Square

Step 3: *Calculate the Pearson Square (utilizing the percentage from Step 2).*

Utilize the Pearson Square method in order to determine the pounds of hay and grain needed to provide the correct percentage of crude protein. The tables below provide necessary nutrient information. Use the animal's total daily intake from Step 1 when determining the specific amounts of hay and grain.

Forage analysis

DE:	0.96 Mcal/lb
CP:	9%
Ca:	0.40%
P:	0.18%

Grain label**

CP:	14%
C. Fat:	6%
C. Fiber:	10%
Ca:	0.90%
P:	0.50%

**Consult Table 10.1 in Lab 10 to determine DE*

Step 4: *Analyze the diet.*

Use the chart below along with the amounts of hay and grain to determine whether the horse's requirements for DE, Ca, and P are met. Since the ration is balanced for crude protein, it's not necessary to complete the protein analysis. (Consult NRC, 2007, pp. 298–299 for DE, Ca, and P requirements.)

Feed	As Fed	DM		DE		CP		Ca		P	
	lb	%	lb	Mcal/lb	Mcal	%	lb	%	lb	%	lb
Hay											
Grain											
Total											
Convert to g								g		g	g
Required:								g		g	g
Difference (+/−):								g		g	g

Laboratory 12
CORRECTING NUTRIENT DEFICIENCIES IN A RATION

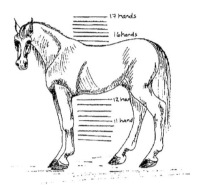

Source: Rachel Monticelli-Turner.

NOTES:

Introduction:

Nutrient deficits may appear in diets, especially in regards to growing animals or those with higher nutrient requirements such as working horses or lactating mares. This laboratory exercise offers a method to correct nutrient deficiencies in horse rations.

Objectives:

When finished with the material from this lab, the student should be able to:

1. Perform "lack divided by gain" to adjust nutrient deficits in the diet.
2. Formulate some guidelines regarding feeding young horses and horses that are under heavy exercise.

Questions for further discussion:

1. Due to soil content, are there any regions of the United States where horses are more likely to be deficient in one nutrient than another?
2. What are potential symptoms caused by nutrient deficiencies?

Manual of Equine Nutrition and Feeding Management, First Edition.
Carol Z. Buckhout and Barbara E. Lindberg.
© 2022 John Wiley & Sons, Inc. Published 2022 by John Wiley & Sons, Inc.
Companion website: www.wiley.com/go/buckhout/manual

NOTES:

Correcting Deficiencies: Lack Divided by Gain

There are times when a nutrient deficit may be revealed from a ration evaluation. This is particularly true for a growing horse, a lactating mare, or for a horse that is being heavily exercised. Depending on the quality and quantity of feed used, any of the major nutrients may be lacking, including digestible energy, crude protein, or the various minerals or vitamins.

In situations with a nutrient deficiency, one needs to determine how much of an additional feed or supplement to add to the horse's diet to correct the deficiency. One method to use is represented by the following equation:

$$\frac{\text{Lack (of specific nutrient)}}{\text{Gain (in nutrient of new feed)}} = \text{Amount of new feed to add}$$

Example: A yearling horse, estimated mature weight of 1100 pounds, is fed 12 pounds of a mixed grass hay and 4 pounds of a pelleted commercial grain per day. The analyses of the hay and grain are listed below. All values listed are on an as sampled basis. The ration analysis may also be done on an as sampled basis. Using the chart and the appropriate NRC (2007) table of daily nutrient requirements, determine whether the horse's daily nutrient requirements are being met.

	Mixed Grass Hay	Pelleted Grain
DM:	90%	90%
DE:	0.77 Mcal/lb	1.45 Mcal/lb
CP:	7.8%	12%
Ca:	0.49%	1.0% (min.)
P:	0.18%	0.55% (min.)

Feed	As Fed	DE		CP		Ca		P	
	lb	Mcal/lb	Mcal	%	lb	%	lb	%	lb
Mixed Hay									
Grain									
Total									
Convert to g					g		g		g
Required:					g		g		g
Difference (+/−):					g		g		g

Do any nutrient deficiencies exist? If so, which nutrients and what is the amount of the deficiency?

The horse in this example may be deficient in both digestible energy and crude protein. This would not be acceptable, especially for a growing horse. Assume there is some second cutting hay available that may be added to the horse's diet. A forage analysis for second cutting hay is provided below. Use the lack divided by gain method to determine how much second cutting hay may be needed. Correct for DE deficiency first and then determine whether other nutrient deficiencies still exist.

Forage Analysis: Second Cutting

DM: 88%

DE: 1.1 Mcal/lb

CP: 12%

Ca: 1.2% (min.)

P: 0.25% (min.)

$$\frac{\text{Lack in DE :}}{\begin{array}{c}\text{Gain in DE}\\\text{from 2nd cutting}\end{array}} = \frac{\boxed{}\ \text{Mcal}}{\boxed{}\ \text{Mcal / lb}} = \boxed{}\ \text{lb 2nd cutting}$$

Feed	As Fed	DE		CP		Ca		P	
	lb	Mcal/lb	Mcal	%	lb	%	lb	%	lb
Mixed Hay									
2nd cut									
Grain									
Total		███		███		███		███	
Convert to g		███			g	███	g		g
Required:					g	███	g	███	g
Difference (+/−):		███	███	███	g	███	g	███	g

It's possible that a crude protein deficiency still exists. If this is the case, one might add some high protein pellets to the horse's diet. Assume there are such pellets available and that they provide 25% crude protein. Use the lack divided by gain method to determine the amount of high protein pellets that need to be added to the grain mix. (Be careful of the units used for this part.)

Lack in CP: $\boxed{}$ g   = $\boxed{}$ g or $\boxed{}$ lb or $\boxed{}$ oz

Gain from Protein Pellets*: $\boxed{}$

*Convert % to a decimal form

With the addition of the protein pellets does the horse receive its daily nutrient requirements? _____

Supplemental Activity
APPLYING LACK/GAIN CONCEPT TO ACTUAL HORSES

Materials:

- Ration evaluation of assigned horse(s)
- Access to information about various feeds and supplements available at the feed store

Objective:

To have students apply the lack/gain concept to their assigned horse(s).

Activity:

1. Determine if assigned horse(s) have any deficiencies expressed in their ration analyses.

2. Select a feed or supplement that would be appropriate to add to the horse's diet, if any.

3. Use the lack/gain concept to determine how much of the feed would be needed to add to the horse's diet, if any.

4. Did the feed selected provide the cheapest way of meeting the horse's requirements?

5. If assigned horse(s) did not have any deficiencies, is there a more cost effective feed that still meets all of their requirements?

Note: Higher-quality feeds that meet all of a horse's requirements may actually cost less than using their cheaper and lower quality counterparts.

Reference:

National Research Council. (2007). *Nutrient Requirements of Horses* (6th ed.). Washington: The National Academies Press.

Name_____

Lab Section_____

Laboratory Assignment 12
ADJUSTING FOR NUTRIENT DEFICIENCIES

1.   A 24-month-old horse with an estimated mature weight of 600 kg is exercised lightly. It receives a diet of 20 pounds of first cutting hay and 6 pounds of Scholar Horse Feed. The analyses for both the first cutting hay and the Scholar Horse Feed are included with this lab assignment.

   a.   Using the chart provided, evaluate this horse's ration to determine whether the first cutting hay and Scholar Horse Feed provide adequate levels of nutrients to meet its daily nutrient requirements. Use the appropriate chart of daily nutrient requirements from the NRC (2007). The evaluation may be done on an as sampled basis.

   b.   If nutrient deficits occur, use the lack divided by gain method to determine the amount of second cutting hay that should be added to the horse's diet. A forage analysis is provided for the second cutting hay. Correct for a DE deficiency first and determine whether all other nutrient deficiencies are corrected as a result of adding the second cutting to the horse's diet.

Feed	As Fed	DE		CP		Ca		P	
	lb	Mcal/lb	Mcal	%	lb	%	lb	%	lb
1st cut									
Scholar									
Total									
Convert to g					g		g		g
Required:					g		g		g
Difference (+/−):					g		g		g

Lack in DE: _____ Mcal   =   _____ lb 2nd cutting

Gain in DE from 2nd cutting: _____ Mcal/lb

Feed	As Fed	DE		CP		Ca		P	
	lb	Mcal/lb	Mcal	%	lb	%	lb	%	lb
1st cut									
Scholar									
2nd cut									
Total									
Convert to g					g		g		g
Required:					g		g		g
Difference (+/−):					g		g		g

Does a CP deficiency exist? _____ If yes, use *lack divided by gain* to determine the amount (in ounces) of high protein pellets (25% CP) that would need to be added.

2. A 1320 pound Thoroughbred brood mare is in her first month of lactation. She is currently fed 4 flakes of first cutting and 4 flakes of second cutting hay (each flake weighs 3.5 pounds) and 6 pounds of Scholar Horse Feed. Evaluate the mare's diet. If nutrient deficiencies occur, use the lack over gain method to determine the amount of additional Brood Mare Feed that should be added to correct for deficiencies. Remember to correct for a possible DE deficiency first. The nutrient analyses for the first and second cutting hays, the Scholar Horse Feed, and the Brood Mare Feed are all provided.

Feed	As Fed	DE		CP		Ca		P	
	lb	Mcal/lb	Mcal	%	lb	%	lb	%	lb
1st cut									
2nd cut									
Scholar									
Total									
Convert to g					g		g		g
Required:					g		g		g
Difference (+/−):					g		g		g

Lack in DE: _____ Mcal = _____ lb Brood Mare Feed

Gain in DE from Brood Mare Feed: _____ Mcal/lb

Feed	As Fed	DE		CP		Ca		P	
	lb	Mcal/lb	Mcal	%	lb	%	lb	%	lb
1st cut									
2nd cut									
Scholar									
B'mare									
Total									
Convert to g					g		g		g
Required:					g		g		g
Difference (+/−):					g		g		g

Does a CP deficiency exist? _____ If yes, use *lack divided by gain* to determine the amount (in ounces) of high protein pellets (25% CP) that would need to be added.

3. A 500 kilogram gelding is exercised at the heavy level. His owners have requested that his ration be evaluated as he appears to be losing weight. He is currently fed 20 pounds of first cutting hay and 6 pounds of Manetain Horse Feed. Using the information provided by the appropriate forage analysis and feed label, evaluate this gelding's diet. Use the appropriate table of daily nutrient requirements from NRC (2007). If a nutrient deficiency occurs, determine the amount of Scholar Horse Feed to add to the gelding's diet using the lack divided by gain method.

Feed	As Fed	DE		CP		Ca		P	
	lb	Mcal/lb	Mcal	%	lb	%	lb	%	lb
1st cut									
Manetain									
Total									
Convert to g					g		g		g
Required:					g		g		g
Difference (+/−):					g		g		g

Lack in DE: _____ Mcal   =   _____ lb Scholar Feed

Gain in DE from Scholar Horse Feed: _____ Mcal/lb

Feed	As Fed	DE		CP		Ca		P	
	lb	Mcal/lb	Mcal	%	lb	%	lb	%	lb
1st cut									
Manetain									
Scholar									
Total									
Convert to g					g		g		g
Required:					g		g		g
Difference (+/−):					g		g		g

Does a CP deficiency exist? _____ If yes, use *lack divided by gain* to determine the amount (in ounces) of high protein pellets (25% CP) that would need to be added. Check the amounts of Ca and P as well as the ratio of Ca to P that the horse receives.

Description 1: FIRST CUTTING

Description 2:

Statement ID:

	%	As Sampled	%	Dry Matter
% Moisture		8.3		
% Dry Matter		91.7		

		As Sampled		Dry Matter
Digestible Energy (DE) Mcal/lb		0.85		0.93

	%	g/lb.	%	g/lb.
Crude Protein	6.5	29.3	7.1	32.0
Estimated Lysine	.22	1.0	.25	1.1
Lignin	7.2	32.9	7.9	35.8
Acid Detergent Fiber (ADF)	39.3	178.4	42.9	194.5
Neutral Detergent Fiber (NDF)	59.2	268.4	64.6	292.8
%WSC (Water Sol. Carbs.)	11.4	51.8	12.5	56.5
ESC (Simple Sugars)	7.2	32.8	7.9	35.8
Starch	1.3	6.0	1.4	6.5
Non-Structural Carb. (NSC)	18.0	81.8	19.7	89.3
Non-Fiber Carb (NFC)	19.8	10.3	21.9	19.2
Crude Fat	1.9	8.5	2.1	9.3
Ash	6.1	27.7	6.7	30.3

	%	g/lb.	%	g/lb.
Calcium	.68	3.09	.74	3.37
Phosphorus	.12	.54	.13	.59
Magnesium	.10	.45	.11	.49
Potassium	1.07	7.71	1.85	8.41
Sodium	.004	.017	.004	.019

	ppm	mg/lb.	ppm	mg/lb.
Iron	90	41	98	45
Zinc	14	6	15	7
Copper	7	3	8	3
Manganese	59	27	64	29
Molybdenum	.62	.28	.68	.31

Description 1: SECOND CUTTING

Description 2:

Statement ID:

% Moisture		10.0		
% Dry Matter		90.1		
		As Sampled		**Dry Matter**
Digestible Energy (DE) Mcal/lb		0.94		1.04
	%	**g/lb.**	**%**	**g/lb.**
Crude Protein	12.4	56.3	13.8	62.5
Estimated Lysine	.58	2.6	.65	2.9
Lignin	7.0	31.9	7.8	35.4
Acid Detergent Fiber (ADF)	32.4	146.8	36.0	163.1
Neutral Detergent Fiber (NDF)	48.0	217.7	53.3	241.7
%WSC (Water Sol. Carbs.)	10.2	46.5	11.4	51.6
ESC (Simple Sugars)	8.4	38.2	9.4	42.4
Starch	.2	1.1	.3	1.2
Non-Structural Carb. (NSC)	8.7	39.3	9.6	43.6
Non-Fiber Carb (NFC)	20.5	93.0	22.8	103.2
Crude Fat	2.7	12.1	3.0	13.4
Ash	6.5	29.5	7.2	32.7

	%	**g/lb.**	**%**	**g/lb.**
Calcium	1.04	4.72	1.16	5.25
Phosphorus	.19	.85	.21	.94
Magnesium	.19	.85	.21	.94
Potassium	1.88	8.54	2.09	9.48
Sodium	.004	.017	.004	.019

	ppm	**mg/lb.**	**ppm**	**mg/lb.**
Iron	74	34	82	37
Zinc	21	10	24	11
Copper	8	4	9	4
Manganese	35	16	39	18
Molybdenum	.44	.20	.49	.22

Scholar Horse Feed

This feed was designed to be fed to the average school horse.

Guaranteed Analysis:

Crude Protein	Min	13.00	%			
Crude Fat	Min	6.00	%			
Crude Fiber	Max	8.00	%			
Calcium	Min	1.00	%	Max	1.20	%
Phosphorus	Min	0.85	%			
Copper	Min	51.00	PPM			
Selenium	Min	0.70	PPM			
Zinc	Min	159.00	PPM			
Vitamin A	Min	3985.30	IU/LB			

Ingredients:

Processed Grain By-Products, Grain Products, Roughage Products, Forage Products, Soybean Meal, Calcium Carbonate, Molasses Products, Plant Protein Products, Salt, Lysine, Methionine Supplement, Natural and Artificial Preservatives, Potassium Chloride, Sodium Selenite, Primaiac, L-Threonine, Zinc Sulfate, Natural & Artificial Flavors added, Copper Sulfate, Selenium Yeast, Selenium, Folic Acid, Zinc Amino Acid Complex, Manganese Supplement, Riboflavin Supplement, Biotin, Thiamine Supplement, Vitamin E Supplement, Vitamin D3 Supplement, Vitamin B12 Supplement, Magnesium Oxide, Cobalt Carbonate, Ferrous Sulfate, Manganese Sulfate, Copper Chloride, Zinc Oxide

***Warning: Do not fed to sheep because it contains supplemental copper.

Product Code: 15638752_THY
Net Wt. 50 LB

Manufactured by:
Scholar Horse Feeds: A Smart Decision
Main Office
Cazenovia, NY, 13035

Lot: 008

Figure 12.1 Feed label example. *Source: Sara Tanner Mastellar.*

Brood Mare Feed

Designed specifically for broodmares.

Guaranteed Analysis:

Crude Protein	Min	16.0	%		
Crude Fat	Min	6.0	%		
Crude Fiber	Max	8.0	%		
Calcium	Min	0.65	%	Max	1.15 %
Phosphorus	Min	0.70	%		
Copper	Min	48.00	PPM		
Manganese	Min	120.50	PPM		
Selenium	Min	0.50	PPM		
Zinc	Min	145.00	PPM		
Vitamin A	Min	5,000.00	IU/lb		

Ingredients:

Steam Crimped Oats, Steam Flaked Corn, Steam Flaked Barley, Wheat Middlings, Soybean Meal, Ground Corn, Dehydrated Alfalfa Meal, Rice Bran, Dried Beet Pulp, Yeast Culture, Corn Distillers Dried Grains, Cane Molasses, Salt, Vegetable Oil, Calcium Carbonate, Monocalcium Phosphate, DL-Methionine, L-Lysine Monohydrochloride, Zinc Sulfate, Copper Sulfate, Manganese Sulfate, Copper Proteinate, Manganese Proteinate, Calcium Propionate, Cobalt Carbonate, Calcium Iodate, Ferrous Sulfate, Sodium Selenite, Selenium Yeast, Vitamin E Supplement, Vitamin A Supplement, Vitamin D3 Supplement, Choline Chloride, Riboflavin, Niacin, Folic Acid, Biotin, Vitamin B12 Supplement, Thiamine Mononitrate, Pyridoxine Hydrochloride, Menadione Sodium Bisulfite Complex (Source of Vitamin K Activity), Oat Mill By-product, Brewers Dried Yeast L-Ascorbyl-2- Polyphosphate (Source of Vitamin C), Yucca Schidigera Extract

***Warning: Do not feed to sheep. Contains supplemental copper.

Product Code: 1943_BOX
Net Wt. 50 LB
Manufactured by:
College Feeds: A Smart Decision
Main Office
Cazenovia, NY, 13035

Lot: 009

Figure 12.2 Feed label example. Source: Sara Tanner Mastellar.

Manetain

This feed was designed to be used to maintain adult horses.

Guaranteed Analysis:

Crude Protein	Min	10.0	%		
Crude Fat	Min	4.0	%		
Crude Fiber	Max	10.00	%		
Calcium	Min	0.65	%	Max	1.05 %
Phosphorus	Min	0.50	%		
Copper	Min	34.00	PPM		
Manganese	Min	108.50	PPM		
Selenium	Min	0.40	PPM		
Zinc	Min	120.00	PPM		
Vitamin A	Min	5,000.00	IU/lb		

Ingredients:

Steam Flaked Corn, Coarse Cracked Corn, Steam Crimped Oats, Cane Molasses, Wheat Middlings, Soybean Hulls, Ground Corn, Vegetable Oil, Salt, Calcium Carbonate, Calcium Sulfate, Monocalcium Phosphate, Zinc Sulfate, Copper Sulfate, Manganese Sulfate, Copper Proteinate, Manganese Proteinate, Calcium Propionate, Cobalt Carbonate, Calcium Iodate, Ferrous Sulfate, Sodium Selenite, Selenium Yeast, Vitamin E Supplement, Vitamin A Supplement, Vitamin D3 Supplement, Choline Chloride, Riboflavin, Niacin, Folic Acid, Biotin, Vitamin B12 Supplement, Thiamine Mononitrate, Pyridoxine Hydrochloride, Menadione Sodium Bisulfite Complex (Source of Vitamin K Activity), Oat Mill By-product, L-Ascorbyl-2-Polyphosphate (Source of Vitamin C), DL-Methionine

***Warning: Do not feed to sheep because it contains supplemental copper.

Product Code: 8675309_JT2
Net Wt. 50 LB
Manufactured by:
College Feeds: A Smart Decision
Main Office
Cazenovia, NY, 13035

Lot: 006

Figure 12.3 Feed label example. Source: Sara Tanner Mastellar.

Laboratory 13
DETERMINING THE COST OF FEEDING

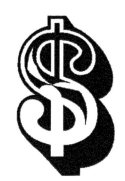

Source: Rachel Monticelli-Turner.

Introduction:

There are numerous costs associated with keeping horses, and feed costs are among the most significant. The purpose of this lab is to identify monthly feeding expenses and to determine ways to minimize these expenses.

Objectives:

When finished with this lab, the student should be able to:

1. Determine the annual expenses of feeding a horse.
2. Understand the variables that can impact feed expenses.
3. Evaluate feeds on a cost per nutrient basis.

Question for further discussion:

1. What are suggestions for minimizing feeding expenses?

General overview:

Numerous factors affect feed costs with two of the most significant factors being climate and location. Seasons with extremes in weather will affect growing and harvesting conditions. When crop yields are low, feed prices will increase. As rural agricultural areas become more populated, fields that once produced quality forages or grains may no longer be in production. Livestock owners in these areas may have to purchase their feeds from other locations. Transportation expenses add to the costs of non-locally grown feeds. Positive relationships with local growers and feed dealers are helpful in the planning and budgeting process in regards to this major equine expense.

Feeds can also be evaluated on their price per nutrient. Energy and protein are the two most popular nutrients used in this evaluation process. Determining the price of a feed based on energy or protein content can be useful in making decisions regarding the most economical purchase. This may be referred to as determining the least cost feed. An example is provided in the next section.

Manual of Equine Nutrition and Feeding Management, First Edition.
Carol Z. Buckhout and Barbara E. Lindberg.
© 2022 John Wiley & Sons, Inc. Published 2022 by John Wiley & Sons, Inc.
Companion website: www.wiley.com/go/buckhout/manual

NOTES:

Determining the least cost of two forages based on digestible energy (Lewis, 1996, pp. 140):

One would need to know the nutrient profile of two different forages from a forage analysis. It would be necessary to determine that energy was the key nutrient to evaluate for a least cost basis. Follow the example below:

	Forage 1:	Forage 2:
DE:	0.8 Mcal/lb	1.0 Mcal/lb
CP:	8.5%	10%
Cost:	$120/ton	$140/ton

While Forage 1 appears to be the better deal, let's compare the forages based on digestible energy:

Forage 1: $120 ÷ (0.8 Mcal × 2000 lb/ton) = $150 / 2000 Mcal

Forage 2 : $140 ÷ (1 Mcal × 2000 lb/ton) = $140 / 2000 Mcal

Therefore even though Feed 1 is less expensive per ton, Feed 2 is more economical based on price per unit of energy.

Carrying this one step farther, the digestible energy requirement for a 500 kg average maintenance horse is 16.7 Mcal of DE (NRC, 2007 pp. 298). To determine the daily cost of Forage 1 versus Forage 2 would be as follows:

Forage 1:
16.7 Mcal / horse / day ÷ 0.8 Mcal / lb = 20.87 lb Forage 1 / horse / day
$\left(20.87 \text{ lb Forage 1 / horse / day} \times \$120 / \text{ton Forage 1}\right) \div 2000 \text{ lb / ton} = \$1.25 / \text{horse / day}$

Forage 2:
16.7 Mcal / horse / day ÷ 1.0 Mcal / lb = 16.7 lb Forage 2 / horse / day
$\left(16.7 \text{ lb Forage 2 / horse / day} \times \$140 / \text{ton Forage 2}\right) \div 2000 \text{ lb / ton} = \$1.16 / \text{horse / day}$

Assuming that the horse is fed hay to meet its daily energy requirement, Forage 2 would be the more economical feed to use as the horse would require less per day (16.7 lb of Forage 2 versus. 20.87 lb of Forage 1). One would round both of these numbers up to account for a certain amount of waste associated with feeding hay. It would also be necessary to determine that the horse's requirements for protein, minerals, and vitamins were also provided for by the forages being used.

Determining the least cost of two concentrate mixes based on crude protein: (Lewis, 1996, pp. 140–141)

The price of commercial concentrates is partially determined by the crude protein content. Determining the price per pound of protein could help in the process to determine which concentrate to purchase. Review the example below:

Concentrate 1:		Concentrate 2:	
Crude Protein:	12%	Crude Protein:	14%
Crude Fat:	6%	Crude Fat:	6%
Crude Fiber:	8%	Crude Fiber:	8%
Price/50 lb:	$11.99	Price/50 lb:	$12.99

1. Determine the price per pound of each feed:
   a. **Concentrate 1:** $11.99 ÷ 50 lb = $0.24/lb
   b. **Concentrate 2:** $12.99 ÷ 50 lb = $0.25/lb
2. Divide price per pound by percent protein:
   a. **Concentrate 1:** 0.24 ÷ 0.12 = $2.00 per pound of crude protein
   b. **Concentrate 2:** 0.25 ÷ 0.14 = $1.78 per pound of crude protein

Explanation: Although Concentrate 2 is more expensive than Concentrate 1, its higher percentage of protein makes its price per pound of protein less than Concentrate 1. An owner with a horse that has a relatively high protein requirement, such as a growing horse or a lactating mare, could benefit economically by being fed Concentrate 2 instead of Concentrate 1. The overall amount of concentrate needed to be fed would be less with Concentrate 2.

NOTES:

References:

Lewis, L. (1996). *Feeding and Care of the Horse* (2nd ed.). Media, PA: Lippincott, Williams and Wilkens.

National Research Council. (2007). *Nutrient Requirements of Horses* (6th ed.). Washington: The National Academies Press.

Supplemental Activity
MINIMIZING FEEDING COSTS FOR AN ASSIGNED HORSE

Materials:

- Ration analysis for an assigned horse
- Access to current feed costs
- Access to information and prices for different feeds and supplements available from a local feed store

Objective:

To have students formulate a ration for a horse in their care with the goal of minimizing costs without compromising nutrients.

Activity:

1. Determine the cost of feeding an assigned horse its current ration for one year.

2. Referring to the ration analysis for the assigned horse and information gathered from a local feed store determine whether there are less expensive feeds to use. This may involve a new ration analysis.

3. Determine the cost of feeding the assigned horse the newly formulated ration for one year.

4. How much money could be saved on an annual basis by switching to this new ration?

Note: You will not need as much of some higher-quality feeds to meet all of a horse's requirements and may actually end up saving money by using them instead of their cheaper and lower quality counterparts.

NOTES:

Name_____

Lab Section_____

Laboratory 13 Assignment
DETERMINING THE COST OF FEEDING

1. Having an appreciation for the costs associated with feeding horses is important for horse owners. In each of the following situations determine the potential annual feeding expenses. Please show your calculations.

    a. A 1200 lb performance horse that receives 20 pounds of hay and 8 pounds of grain daily. The hay is priced at $3.50/bale with an average weight/bale of 50 pounds. The price of the grain is $13.99 for a 50 pound bag. In addition, it receives a vitamin/mineral supplement that costs $27.99 for 5 pounds which is intended to last for 160 days.

b. A 1400 pound performance horse that receives 18 pounds of first cutting hay, 8 pounds of second cutting hay and 10 pounds of grain daily. The price of the first cutting hay is $4.00 per bale with a bale weighing 60 pounds on average; the price of the second cutting hay is $5.00 per bale with a bale weighing 50 pounds on average and the price of the grain is $12.49 for a 50 pound bag. The horse also receives an oral joint supplement which costs $0.85/day.

c. A 950 pound two-year-old filly has an estimated mature weight of 1100 pounds. She is already being exercised at a light level of exercise and is being fed 12 pounds of first cutting hay, 6 pounds of second cutting hay and 6 pounds of grain daily. In six months, her grain intake will increase to 8 pounds per day. The first cutting hay costs $5.00/bale with an average weight per bale of 80 pounds; the second cutting hay costs $5.50/bale with an average weight of 60 pounds per bale and the grain costs $14.50 per 50 pound bag.

d. Summarize your observations about feeding expenses for horses.

2. A hay supplier has located two different types of hay, one that is a mostly grass first cutting hay and another that is a mixed grass and legume second cutting hay. Their analyses are listed below. Please complete the series of questions that follow:

Cost/ton:	$100.00	$115.00
DE:	0.88 Mcal/lb	1.1 Mcal/lb
CP:	8.1%	12.5%
Ca:	0.38%	1.1%
P:	0.23%	0.3%

a. What is the price per 2000 Mcal of digestible energy for each of the forages? Please show calculations.

b. Compare the daily potential expense of feeding each type of forage to an 1100 pound performance horse exercised at moderate activity. How would you determine the amount of each hay to use? Show your calculations for this and summarize your findings. Which hay would you recommend?

3. Evaluate two different concentrate mixes that are recommended for performance horses. The guaranteed analysis of each feed is listed below. Calculate the price per pound of protein for each feed. Suggest a situation that each concentrate could be used in a certain horse's diet.

	Concentrate 1:	Concentrate 2:
Crude Protein:	12%	16%
Crude Fat:	6%	7%
Crude Fiber:	8%	10%
Price/50 lb:	$12.99	$14.49

4. You have a boarding facility and are buying hay to feed your horses throughout the year. You are considering hay from two vendors. The first vendor sells hay by the truckload (40 bales weighing 50 lb each) for $150 per truckload. The forage analysis states that the DE for this hay is 0.80 Mcal per lb. The second vendor sells hay by the wagon (200 bales weighing 40 lb each) for $600 a wagon. This hay was analyzed and found to have 0.85 Mcal per lb. Determine which hay is the best value per Mcal of DE.

Challenge question:

1. Determine the most economical forage to purchase based on price per pound of protein. Please show calculations used to determine this.

Forage A:

$150/ton

Crude protein: 7.8%

Forage B:

$180/ton

Crude protein: 9.0%

Forage C:

$210/ton

Crude Protein: 13%

INDEX

A

absorption 1, 20, 21

Acid Detergent Fiber (ADF) 46, 47

acre 45, 49, 55

activated trypsin enzyme 16

additives 85, 86, 93, 96,

aging a horse by its teeth 5

alfalfa 24, 28, 48, 58, 68

alfalfa cubes 25

alfalfa meal 93

algebraic equation 88

almond hulls 93

alsike clover 24, 29, 32, 68

alveolus 3

amino acids 16

amylase 16

antibiotic feed additives 96

antioxidants 96

anus 14

apex of cecum 11, 12

as fed/as sampled basis 85, 87–89, 91, 93, 97, 98, 101, 102, 105, 106, 129, 130, 136, 139, 140, 152

Association of American Feed Control Officials (AAFCO) 132

Avena sativa 75

B

bahia grass 24, 69

bale 47, 57, 58, 60–62, 89

bar 3 *see also* diastema

barley 24, 76, 83

barley hay 58

base of cecum 11–13

bedding 24, 30, 31

beet pulp 73, 86

beet, sugar pulp (unmolassed) 93

bermuda grass 24, 69

bile 15, 16

birdsfoot trefoil 24, 30, 58, 68

bit 4

bitter 7

black walnut 31

blister beetle 31

blood sugar regulation 15

bluegrass 24, 26, 48, 58, 62, 69

bluestem 24

body condition scoring 71, 73

body of the cecum 11

body weight 57, 63, 67, 112, 115, 117, 118, 124, 127, 129, 130, 139, 140, 151

bone meal 86

botulism 31

brachyodont 4

bracken fern 34

brewer's grains 93

bridle teeth 3 *see also* canine

brome grass 24, 58, 62, 69

Bromus inermis 27

buccal points 6

burdocks 30, 48

buttercups 34, 48

by-product 71, 72, 79, 85, 86, 93–95

C

calcium (Ca) 46, 102, 103, 106, 107, 110, 112, 115, 117, 122–124, 129, 130, 136

calories (c) 46, 110, 111

Manual of Equine Nutrition and Feeding Management, First Edition.
Carol Z. Buckhout and Barbara E. Lindberg.
© 2022 John Wiley & Sons, Inc. Published 2022 by John Wiley & Sons, Inc.
Companion website: www.wiley.com/go/buckhout/manual